Praise for The A

"Jon Anderson is one of my favorite people! I loved reading his new book, *The Acceptance*. It was a fun read and filled with insightful thoughts and great wisdom. His wit, humor, and humility let you know he is a fellow struggler on this journey to experience our most important human relationships."

Carl Caton – Founder/President – The San Antonio Marriage Initiative

"Everyone knows deep down that strong, healthy relationships are hard work. But most people don't know what that hard work actually looks like. This is why you need to read *The Acceptance!* Jon Anderson has decades of personal and professional experience in helping couples practice the principles of true love and intimacy. And one of the most difficult principles to practice is acceptance.

Full of research, real life stories, and solid biblical truth, *The Acceptance* will inspire and equip you to truly love well. I highly recommend this book for couples of all ages and stages."

Jonathan Daugherty – Founder & President – Be Broken

"Jon Anderson has managed to take his life's work and study as a counselor and therapist and make it easy to understand and apply. Jon's voice as a writer cuts through all the junk and jargon that so often fills the courses, books, and seminars on relationships. *The Acceptance* explains what is going on in our relationships and provides practices that real people can walk out in real life in pursuit of the relationships we all want and need."

Dr. Darrell Smith – Author of "Faith Lies"

"*The Acceptance* would have been enormously helpful through a number of challenging seasons my wife and I have navigated across our 62 years of marriage. It is written in a refreshing style and is based on sound research. More importantly it grows out of 25 years of professional experience, serving over 3000 couples directly (tens of thousands indirectly) – plus 34 years of living inside a 'real life' marriage."

**Dr. Lynn Anderson – Author of "They Smell Like Sheep",
"Talking Back to God", and "The Shepherd's Song"**

More Praise for The Acceptance

"Symphonically weaving story-telling, scientific research, and professional experiences, Jon Anderson discover the tools necessary for authentic marriages. Couples cultivating their own long-term health and happiness may not be needing to read The Acceptance, but they surely will be wanting to read it."

Dr. Don Lucas – Author of "Being: Your Happiness, Pleasure and Contentment",
Host of YouTube Channel "5MIWeekly"

"Jon and his family have been committed to strengthening marriages and family as long as I've known him, and that has been over 20 years. His advice is based on scripture in real world marriages."

David Robinson - NBA MVP and Champion, Founder of the Carver Academy

"Articulate, compassionate and effective, are characteristics of my friend, colleague, and advocate for healthy, happy relationships. Blessings to all who practice the principles laid out in *The Acceptance!*"

Dr. Patricia Adams – Clinical Director/CEO – Zeitgeist Wellness Group

"Jon Anderson really understands how to help marriages. From the home needing a tune-up to the family needing an overhaul, Jon can help. I would trust him with any challenge or concern. He is a terrific resource. And, even more, he is a dear friend."

Max Lucado – New York Times Bestselling Author

"Hands down, you can trust Jon's work and *The Acceptance*! Using real stories and clear research, Jon lays a reliable path for any couple to be one another's first choice. Practical tools also provide tangible ways to lead any couple toward hope and a thriving marriage relationship. For nearly married couples to veterans, Danny and I are delighted to add *The Acceptance* to our arsenal of marriage resources."

Anna Panter – Coufounder of Marriage Strong

THE ACCEPTANCE

THE ACCEPTANCE

What Brings And Keeps Lifelong Love

Jon R. Anderson

ELM HILL

A Division of
HarperCollins Christian Publishing

www.elmhillbooks.com

The Acceptance
What Brings And Keeps Lifelong Love

Published in Nashville, Tennessee, by Elm Hill, an imprint of Thomas Nelson. Elm Hill and Thomas Nelson are registered trademarks of HarperCollins Christian Publishing, Inc.

Elm Hill titles may be purchased in bulk for educational, business, fund-raising, or sales promotional use. For information, please e-mail SpecialMarkets@ ThomasNelson.com.

Scripture quotations marked NIV are from the Holy Bible, New International Version˚, NIV˚. Copyright © 1973, 1978, 1984, 2011 by Biblica, Inc.˚ Used by permission of Zondervan. All rights reserved worldwide. www.Zondervan.com. The "NIV" and "New International Version" are trademarks registered in the United States Patent and Trademark Office by Biblica, Inc.˚

Library of Congress Cataloging-in-Publication Data

Library of Congress Control Number: 2019914764

ISBN 978-1-400328178 (Paperback)
ISBN 978-1-400328185 (Hardbound)
ISBN 978-1-400328192 (eBook)

for Landon

TABLE OF CONTENTS

OUR BASIC DRIVE

Our Basic Drive

I have a nephew named Landon. In late 2016, when he was just twenty-two years old, Landon walked out one morning, got some breakfast, and then walked another couple of blocks to a tree which he then climbed up and, using his sweatshirt as a rope, proceeded to hang himself.

By the time he was discovered, he was already brain-dead. On the ambulance ride to the hospital, the EMTs were able to revive his heart but nothing else. Landon wasn't carrying any identification with him that day, so he spent a couple of days on life support until his parents were located. The most heartbreaking and gut-wrenching moment of my life was when I walked into that hospital room to see his lifeless body expanding and contracting, as the ventilator pumped oxygen in and out of his lungs.

Just a few weeks before, I was kayaking down the Guadalupe River with Landon and his uncle Russ. In that moment, Landon was singing joyful songs, as he paddled his kayak slowly along, so loudly that part of me was basking in his joy with a smile, but part of me was a little unnerved because I had not witnessed Landon being anything other than stoic or manic or somewhat distant since he was a boy. I had always liked the challenge of trying to get him to smile, and I considered it a huge success those rare occasions I got a laugh out of him. Now, his dad and I were locked in the most intensely sorrowful embrace I may ever experience.

Landon's battle with schizophrenia had ended.

There's more to tell you about Landon. First, let me tell you about a guy named Maslow.

In 1943, a psychologist named Abraham Maslow wrote a paper called "A Theory of Human Motivation." It described a basic model to explain what motivates us humans to do whatever we are doing, in any circumstance. If you've happened to take a basic psychology course, you will probably remember learning about Maslow's hierarchy of needs, a pyramid-shaped model that illustrates his theory. In my years as a college psychology teacher, I got pretty familiar with this model. For the most part, it is fairly useful. That's probably one big reason why it is still so widely taught and used, more than seventy-five years later. But this popular perspective has blinded us to something that, once you recognize it, will completely change the way you see why people do what they do—how they behave, how they relate, and, even, what motivates us to do anything we do.

It is of the utmost importance that we first take a quick look at this pyramid so that you get a grasp of why the things this book will reveal are so crucial to experiencing lifelong love. Although Maslow and others have tweaked this model over time, here it is in one of its most commonly used forms:

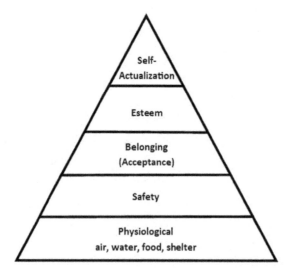

Now, a short explanation:

Each section of the pyramid relies on the sections below it to be reasonably fulfilled, in order for it to matter. So, in order for you to be motivated to find safety, you would first need to have your physical needs (air, water, food, shelter) met. Once you have those things, you begin to be motivated to attain safety. Once you feel relatively safe, you begin to be motivated to belong with, and be accepted by, others. Once you feel relatively accepted, you begin to be motived to acquire esteem. Esteem can also be described as a sense of purpose or status. Once you feel like you have reached a certain degree of esteem, you begin to be motivated toward self-actualization, which may also be described as "striving toward your full potential."

It is important to note that, according to this model, you are not motivated by anything above the stage you are in unless you have obtained the things below your present stage. If you lose something on one of the levels below you, you will no longer be motivated to attain the things above you until you have obtained what it means to be in the stage you are currently in. For example, if I am currently in the middle stage (belonging/acceptance) and then someone cuts off my water supply, I drop down to being only motivated to replace or replenish my water supply.

About a year ago, I was writing a blog article in my study, which has a window looking out onto our street, when I noticed that a truck pulled up with the insignia "San Antonio Water Systems" on the side of it. A man got out, with a long iron tool, and proceeded to turn off my water. At that moment, a sudden feeling of slight panic came over me as I thought about the meeting I had coming up in a couple of hours, and I needed a shower. I went out to ask him how long the water would be shut off, to which he replied, "until you pay your bill."

I had forgotten to pay the water bill! So, I then asked him, "If I were to get online and pay it right now, how long would it be before someone turns it back on?"

To this he replied, "It depends on how backed up we are. Not less than a couple hours but probably before the day is over."

Now panic had just been ratcheted up a notch or two. I ran back in the house, got on line, and paid the bill. But my next step was *not* to continue writing the blog article. Instead, I had to start looking for another place to get a shower before my meeting, which was now about an hour and a half away. The moment before the water department pulled up, I was probably somewhere between "Esteem" and "Self-Actualization." Then I lost one of my physiological needs (water), and nothing else above that stage mattered in the moment.

So, you see why this model is still so widely taught and utilized.

But here is one enormous problem with Maslow's model: Belonging/ Acceptance should be at the very *bottom* of the pyramid! Acceptance matters to us more than survival itself.

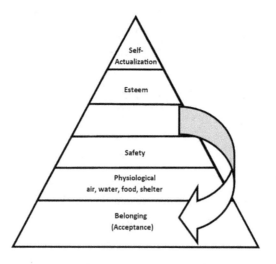

Back to Landon... Landon's father is a successful physician and a partner in a large medical practice. His parents always provided him with all the food, water, shelter, and air that he needed. The first stage of Maslow's hierarchy was never left unfulfilled for Landon, from day one.

As you can imagine, stage two of Maslow's model (Safety) was not an issue for him either. But that third stage "Belonging/Acceptance"[1] had been steadily dissolving as Landon's illness made it increasingly difficult for him to hold a job. Because of schizoaffective-related behaviors, Landon was constantly being misperceived and misunderstood by even his closest relationships, not to mention those in law enforcement and correctional institutions who were, by nature of his erratic behavior, increasingly a part of his life. You see, we can have all the safety and food and shelter and air and water that we could possibly want. But, if we don't feel accepted, or at least have a reasonable amount of hope that we *can* be accepted, we don't even care about living.

By the way, I have never seen parents work so tirelessly to provide their child with feelings of acceptance and belonging, which brings us to another crucial piece to all of this: we desperately want to feel that acceptance from at least one *nonfamily* person as well. In good families, you're going to be loved no matter what. Those of us who grew up in healthy families want more. We want to believe that we can be accepted by someone who doesn't *have* to love us just because we're family. Those without that support system, so much more.

When you begin to see people through this lens, so much more makes sense. Peel back the layers of pretty much any human behavior and you will see it. Why do some strive to be rich? Why do some strive to be famous? Why do some strive to be the life of the party? Why do some strive to be the smartest person in the room? Why do some strive to be the nicest person in the group? Why do some strive to be the most humble or best looking or most athletic or most laid-back or least worrisome or most wise or toughest (badass) or best host or most artistic or coolest or most loving or most serving or most faithful or most joyful or most

---

[1] The word "belonging" is used in most versions of Maslow pyramid. I choose to use the word "acceptance" instead because, at least in my understanding of the two terms, it more clearly represents what I believe Maslow and his model are attempting to convey. For example, I can *belong* to a club because I pay my dues and have a membership card. However, that doesn't mean that the members of the club *accept* me otherwise.

peaceful or kindest or most good or most gentle or most self-controlled or most accepting?

Sometimes the better angels of our nature are riding shotgun to our demons.

Now there may be someone reading this who says to themselves: "None of those are me. I don't strive to be the *mostest* in any category. I just strive to be a good human being." Here's the label you strive for: *best all-around human, at least in my tribe.*

But this isn't about making us feel guilty or wretched. On the contrary, this is how we are wired. We were meant to desire acceptance.

Let's look at it in another way.

From as far back as you may remember, there were two voices at war in your head. One voice said:

Wouldn't it be great if you could find someone who would choose you over everyone else and, even when that person learned pretty much everything there is to know about you—all your bad habits, all the bad things you've done, all of the hurtful things you continue to do, all of your weird emotions, all of your sick thoughts, and so on—and even though they know all that about you, they continue to choose you, over everyone else, for the rest of their life?

That would seem to be the apex of acceptance!
But the other voice says something like this:

Get real! Do you really believe that anyone who knows all that about you would choose you and continue to choose you for the rest of their life? If that person exists, they ain't worth having in the first place. You ain't foolin' no one but yourself!

If you don't have some version of these two voices in your head, you have attained some version of perpetual Nirvana or are an enlightened Zen master or something like that. I want your autograph!

Wait, no. I don't trust you

Why don't I trust you? Because I want to believe that everyone else is at least as messed up as me, which would make me relatively acceptable.

But seriously, I am a counselor by trade and training. So far, I have counseled about 19,500 total hours. If you were to put all my counseling hours back-to-back, it would come out to roughly two years and three months of continuous, twenty-four hours, seven days a week, twelve months a year, working directly with someone who is struggling with something in life.

Wow, I just realized I've screwed up a lot of lives!

Quite often, I will be counseling with someone who thinks they have it all pretty much together. My first question is, "Then why are you here?"

But more than that, these are usually my most dysfunctional clients. And, more tellingly, they are the ones who are most desperately clawing their way into convincing themselves, and usually their spouses, that they are acceptable.

Which they are not.

And, really, neither am I.

And, really, neither are you.

Please hang with me for a moment longer.

This is not about self-loathing. But, if you deserve acceptance, then I ask why?

If your answer is "Because I am a human being, which makes me a child of God," okay, I totally agree. But if there is any other reason, whatsoever, then you and I have issues.

The other day I heard a famous person being interviewed on the radio. This person has had more than one failed marriage, which was part of the conversation. In the interview, this person made a statement that caught my attention in an offhanded way:

"I deserve to be loved."

He wasn't saying it in a way that suggested that anyone who has ever lived deserves to be loved. He was saying it in a way that suggested that certain people deserve to be loved and certain people don't. Not only does that notion ruffle my greasy, dirty feathers, it is, what I would deem, the mindset that is the far-leading contributor to failed relationships (although I will share several close front runners in the following chapters).

Consider this:

Did Adolf Hitler deserve to be loved?
Did Osama bin Laden deserve to be loved?
Did Saddam Hussein deserve to be loved?
Okay, how about these:
Did Lyndon Baines Johnson deserve to be loved?
Did Richard M. Nixon deserve to be loved?
Did Malcolm X deserve to be loved?
Did J. Edgar Hoover deserve to be loved?
Too far from your reality? How about this:
Does George W. Bush deserve to be loved?
Does William J. Clinton deserve to be loved?
Does Donald J. Trump deserve to be loved?
Does Barrack Obama deserve to be loved?
Still too far from your reality?

Does the person down the street who flies the Confederate flag and refuses to let his nineteen-year-old daughter date a black man deserve to be loved?

Does the person next door who came here, knowing that is was illegal, from Central America and doesn't pick up the poop that her dog leaves, every day, on your driveway deserve to be loved?

Maybe this is still too much a part of the media world and not your experience. Let's try something else:

Does the guy who hangs out with you and your friends and acts like a total jerk, on a weekly basis, to everyone around deserve to be loved?

Does the woman who is part of your regular circle of friends and who makes an embarrassing scene every time you are all out in public, and verbally throws everyone under the bus, deserve to be loved?

Okay. Down to the nitty-gritty:

Why does anyone deserve to be loved?

Again, if the answer is because they are human, then I'm down with that. Anything else is just a never-ending, never-winning, always-losing comparison game.

So, a starting point to hope for lifelong love is this: I don't deserve to be loved by my mate, and I will never deserve their love more than they deserve mine.

With that said, I will confess that there are moments when I think to myself, "I deserve her love more than she deserves mine." But the sooner I put that thought in the trash where it belongs, the sooner my life and marriage get back on a good track. When I continue to harbor those thoughts, they begin to grow, and I begin to resent her more and more. That leads me to treating her worse and worse, which leads to her liking me less and less, and the vicious cycle spirals further down into a relationship that becomes more and more unfulfilling.

Acceptance is at the core of what drives us to look for a mate. Acceptance is at the core of what makes us *fall in love*.[2] Acceptance is at the core of that love lasting a lifetime.

---

[2] At this point I am using the term "fall in love" because it is the most common term that our culture uses to describe a universal phenomenon. Many would argue that a person cannot fall out of love because true love does not go away. I would tend to agree with that perspective which is why I will be suggesting another term later in the book. But for now, I will use the terms *fall in love, falling in love, and falling out of love*, since those terms are more widely used and accepted.

THE RELATIONSHIP POOL

The Relationship Pool

Have you ever seen one of those swimming pools that starts off at zero feet deep and then gradually slopes toward the deep end where the water is over your head? Even if you haven't, look at the illustration below. It should prove helpful to understanding the basic dynamics of how we fall in love and how we stay in love or fall out of love.

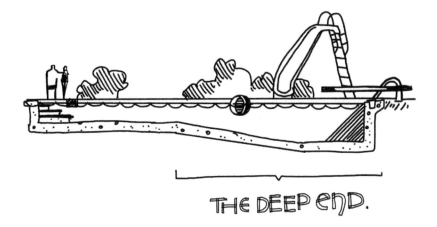

THE DEEP END.

Now, imagine that every relationship that you have, with anyone, is its own pool, laid out just like this one.

The shallow end is the safest part. It's difficult to get hurt in or for someone to hold you under.

The deep end is the most exciting part. It's where all the fun stuff is—the slide, the diving board, and the blob.

Sometimes relationships start off with two people jumping straight into the deep end, especially among younger or less wise or less experienced people. They trust that it's going to be safe and that the other person won't drown them. But those relationships often don't last because one person does something, or fails to do things, which leads the other to decide to get out of the pool all together. Maybe one finds out that the other tends to dunk them every time he or she comes up for air after going off the diving board.

However, for the most part, people tend to start out at the shallow end with the other person, maybe just deep enough to get their toes wet. As they feel safer, they take a step toward deeper waters. But, any time that something happens that gives them a lesser sense of safety, they are going to step backward toward the shallow end.

But first, there is something that happens before either one even decides to give that pool a chance. That thing is called "attraction."

All romantic relationships start off with some sort of attraction. Even though some people will tell me "I wasn't attracted to my spouse at first," there was, nevertheless, some sort of attraction there. It's just that it probably wasn't *sensual* attraction. But there are other types of attraction. So, let's look at the three main types of attraction:

Sensual Attraction

This is the most commonly recognized type of attraction. Sensual attraction refers to one or more of the five senses: sight, sound, smell, taste, and touch. So, when someone says they weren't attracted to their spouse at first, they may be saying that she or he didn't catch their eye. But we often hear people saying things like "I was drawn to his accent," or "when she walked by, her perfume grabbed my attention," or "When he brushed up against me, it was like electricity ran through my body."

We usually don't go around tasting people to see if we might want to date them, so I'll leave that one to your imagination.

Cognitive Attraction

This refers to the way you think about someone. It may be that you like what they are in to or what they do for a living. Maybe it's their basic philosophy of life or the way they think. But cognitive attraction isn't always about similarities. Sometimes we are drawn to something that is totally opposite from ourselves.

When Joanna and I first met, I noticed, right off the bat, that she was extremely conversational and outgoing. I, on the other hand, tend to score on the introverted side of personality assessments. A big part of my attraction to her was that there was something about her that I didn't have. So, someone can be without the things that attract us sensually but still get our attention with how we think about them. By the way, Joanna also has the stunning good looks, providing me with a double dose of attraction to her.

Affective Attraction

Affect refers to the way we feel, emotionally. Someone can be without the attributes that sensually attract us. And, we may not find much about them that cognitively attracts us. But, over time we may feel more and more attracted to him or her because of the way we feel about ourselves when we are around that person. Affective attraction is often the type of attraction that brings two people to start dating each other, who were friends first. In fact, it may well be that the fact they felt safe and comfortable around each other is because neither felt any sort of sensual attraction. But, as time went on, each noticed the ease of the relationship and how it always seemed to be a pleasant experience. By the way, if you become really good at showing acceptance to someone, you can become extremely attractive to him or her, even if you have a face that your own mother can't bear to look at. And, we find many older couples, whose outward appearance has been ravaged by time and gravity, who find each other more attractive than they did forty years ago, simply because they have gotten better and better about making each other feel good about themselves. On the flip side, you see some who seem to get better and better looking with age, while his or her spouse becomes less and less attracted to them because they don't feel accepted by them, thus losing their affective attraction for him or her.

It only takes one of these types of attraction to get things started. But there must be some sort of attraction to get one to be willing to try out the pool with the other:

Sensual attraction
Cognitive attraction
Affective attraction

It should also be noted that it doesn't have to be just one type of attraction. It is often a combination of two of them. If all three are going on, it's likely to be an even stronger attraction.

A few years ago, I was presenting this model at a marriage retreat. Afterward, one of the audience members came up to me and said that it didn't apply to him because he met his wife on a blind date. I asked him if it was *truly* a blind date. Did someone just come up to him and offer to hook him up on a blind date, and he immediately accepted the invitation without finding out more about her? Of course not! Before he accepted, he had some questions: What is she like? Do you have a picture? If not, can you describe what she looks like? What is she in to? What's her history? You gotta at least know if she is married or not, right? Before he was willing to try out the pool, he had to be sure that there was something attractive about her. So, attraction is the first step. We will be coming back to it later, though, because it continues to be important.

So, now the two people have some sort of attraction to each other, so they walk over to the pool together. One takes a step into the water which is, at this part, about an inch deep. He says to her something like "Do you come to this pool often?" The *pickup* line.

You ever notice how much is out there about pickup lines? Pickup lines are huge! I just went to Google and typed in p-i-c. Before I even got to "k," it popped up "pick-up-lines," with, get this, four hundred and sixteen million results.

I couldn't resist clicking on one of those results that said "Funny, cheesy pick-up lines." I have two grown daughters, Abby and Ana, who both live out of town. They and their mom are all very fit and we like to go to the gym together when they visit. One of my favorite ways to fulfill my fatherly duties of embarrassing them in public is to walk up to them after they have done a set of push-ups or something and say a cheesy pickup line to them at a volume where others around can hear. Just found one I'm going to use next time: *Are you my appendix? Because I have a funny feeling in my stomach that makes me think I should take you out.*

By the way, I get off subject a lot. Some people appreciate it, most don't.

Why does a pickup line matter so much? Because… getting the other person to step into the pool next to you all seems to hinge on it. If it's done well, the other person might even take a bigger first step than yourself. If you mess it up, the other person leaves you standing there by yourself, crushed, rejected, shamed… *unaccepted.*

In other words, this process requires *vulnerability*. But the vulnerability is not just on the part of the first person to make a move. If the other person has any desire to try this pool out as well, she also must make herself vulnerable. If she says "I don't know how to swim, but I like swimming pools because they remind me of my favorite movie, *Splash*," well, she has just made herself pretty vulnerable, not just because she has revealed a lack of swimming skills, but she has also revealed that she has horrible taste in movies. (No offense Tom Hanks. You are one of my favorite actors, and my desire to feel accepted has me imagining you reading my book and chuckling to yourself at this point.)

If you didn't even know that Tom Hanks starred in a movie called *Splash*, my point is made.

Or, she could play it safe. When he asks "Do you come to this pool often," she could simply reply with a deadpan "No." If that's the case, it's important to get a visual of the scene at this point. The mutual attraction led them up to the edge of the pool, side by side. Their eyes meet, and he takes a step into the pool as his head is pivoting to keep his eyes locked with hers as he asks her the question. In her first scenario answer, she is taking a step in the same direction as her head is pivoting to maintain eye contact. Now they are again standing side by side, on equal footing. She will now likely follow up her response with a question back to him: "How about you? Do you come to this pool often?" As she is asking this follow-up question, she is now taking another step in the direction of the deep end, indicating to him that she would like for him to be vulnerable as well.

In the other scenario, where she simply replies to his question with "No," she is still standing behind him with her feet dry. He's not going to feel very accepted at this point. If he has a hard time dealing with rejection, or if she just doesn't seem to be worth it *that* much, he will just move on to another pool and/or person. But, if she still seems worth it, his next move is to step back out of the water and try another approach.

So, we have this age-old ritual: she asks a question, he gives an answer; he asks a follow-up question, she gives an answer; she asks a follow-up question, he answers; and so on.

Here's the typical dialogue:

Her: "So, what kind of music do you like?"

Him: "Oh, I like lots of types of music. How about you?"

Her: "Yeah, I like lots of types of music too. What's one of your favorite groups?"

Him: "Well, it depends on the type of music. If it's regular rock, for instance, I can always do some U2. What about you?"

Her: "Well if we're talking about rock 'n' roll, you can't ignore U2, but when I think of rock 'n' roll, I think of more classic old stuff like Led Zeppelin."

Him: "Yeah, Led Zeppelin had some good songs. What do you like better, hip-hop or R&B?"

Her: "I like exercising to hip-hop but if I'm at a wedding, the DJ better have a good smattering of classic R&B mixed in."

Him: "I've been in some crazy line dances at a few weddings."

Her: "Western line dancing is fun!"

That's what they said to each other. Here's what they were thinking, *in italics.*

Her: "So, what kind of music do you like?" *What I really want to know is what he does for a living because, by the way he's dressed, I'm not even sure he has a job.*

Him: "Oh, I like lots of types of music. How about you?" *I've recently been turned onto a K-pop group that is actually really good. Nobody knows it but I have about eighteen of their songs on a playlist safely titled "mom's favorites."*

Her: "Yeah, I like lots of types of music too. What's one of your favorite groups?" *The last time I told a guy how much I like Taylor Swift, he told me to grow up. I'll spin it back to him.*

Him: "Well, it depends on the type of music. If it's regular rock, for instance, I can always do some U2. What about you?" *As far as safe answers go, I just might be a genius.*

Her: "Well if we're talking about rock 'n' roll, you can't ignore U2, but when I think of rock 'n' roll, I think of more classic old stuff like Led Zeppelin." *I want to move on to an artist who didn't turn fifty before I was even born. But, as long as we are here. Wait, why did I blurt out Led Zeppelin? What if he asks me my favorite Led Zeppelin song? Do I even know a Led Zeppelin song? Oh, yeah. "Stairway to Heaven." Whew!*

Him: "Yeah, Led Zeppelin had some good songs. What do you like better, hip-hop or R&B?" *Wait, what if she now asks me what my favorite Led Zeppelin song is? Quick, change genres.*

Her: "I like exercising to hip-hop but if I'm at a wedding, the DJ better have a good smattering of classic R&B mixed in." *Did I just say hip-hop? Who am I? I never say hip-hop. I say rap. Is there a difference? What if he says something like, "but do you like rap as much as hip-hop?" Quick, shift the conversation to another genre. Wait, I just said R&B. Is that the same as soul? Shift to dancing and weddings.*

Him: "I've been in some crazy line dances at a few weddings." *You need to know up front that I don't dance.*

Her: "Western line dancing is fun"! *Wait, is line dancing Western or country? Is there a difference?*

The shear amount of energy of that conversation doesn't seem hardly worth it, not to mention if they spent a ton of time and money setting that moment up! Couldn't we just cut through all the crap and get down to what we really want to know? Can't we just jump into the deep end and find out if there are any "deal breakers" before we spend all this time, money, and energy on two or three or more dates?

I can't tell you how long this ritual of courtship has been going on. I'm sure that in some cultures it's fairly new. But, in some form or fashion, it has been going on for centuries. And, for years, people have been trying to get around it. Take the 1990s, for instance.

Remember speed dating? It was featured in several movies of the the 1990s and early 2000s. Here's how it works: You spend a sum of money, let's say one hundred dollars. You are promised that for your one hundred dollars, you will have twelve dates in two hours. That's one date every ten minutes. What was so appealing about this? Well, you could save a lot of time, money, and energy by cutting past all the fluff and getting down to what really matters. You sat across from someone for ten minutes, and, if things went well, you would exchange phone numbers and call them later that night for a near-in-the-future date where you wouldn't have to talk about all of that superficial stuff and could save the resources it would normally take to get through dates one through four or more. In that ten minutes, you wouldn't waste time talking about music. You would talk about what might be considered "deal breakers":

What are your spiritual or religious views, if any?
Do you want children?
If so, how many and when?
What are your political ideals?

You know… the stuff that really matters to you.

In speed dating, if you heard an answer that was contrary to what you believed, no problem, the date would be over in a few minutes, and you didn't have to go through the grueling process of letting the other person down gently while still making it clear that you never wanted to see him or her again. The ten-minute bell would save you and you could say something like, "Well, I guess our time's up. It was a pleasure getting to know you, and I wish you all the best without myself being, in any sense of the term, a part of your future." No harm, no foul!

So why did speed dating go away, for the most part?

Along comes the Internet—the gigantic on-ramp that would trample speed dating more than a civilization with armored tanks invading a tiny nation that only has bows and arrows. Now, you don't even have to leave your house, much less take a shower. You can spend less than fifty dollars and have the virtual equivalent of ten thousand of those dates simply by submitting a photo, taking a personality assessment, running down a checklist of likes and dislikes, writing a short essay about your fondness for cats (or lack thereof), and hitting "done," and within seconds, *voila*, you have sixty people that it would have taken ten years and four-hundred speed-dating sessions to find. Genius!

Except…

Both speed dating and even sophisticated dating websites leave out a vitally important piece of the courtship process. That piece is the entire shallow end of the pool, that is, what happens from the moment your toes get wet, until you're in over your head. Additionally, the shallow end of the pool is vitally important for maintaining the relationship for years and decades to come. So, let's take a closer look at what's happening at the shallow end.

We start out at the shallow end by making ourselves vulnerable. Okay, it's not profound vulnerability about our deepest thoughts and feelings, at first. But it is, nonetheless, vulnerability. Vulnerability is simply letting others see things about you that, if they reject or ridicule, could leave you hurt. It doesn't hurt as much if someone rejects something superficial about me, like my favorite flavor of ice cream, as it does if they reject the things that matter to me most. Furthermore, the more rejection we experience with someone at superficial levels, the less vulnerable we are going to be when it comes to our more hidden thoughts and feelings. So, whether we realize it or not, the shallow end routine is how we build the trust to go deeper or destroy the trust to be in the pool with that person at all.

I love pretty much all types of food, although I'm not too fond of liver. But let's say, for arguments sake, that I despise Italian food. I'm having one of my first get-to-know-you conversations with someone I'm attracted to. I ask her, "what kind of food do you like?"

She answers, "Oh, Italian is my favorite."

I reply, "Italian?!? How could Italian be anyone's favorite? It's all just a bunch of variations on pasta and red sauce!"

Which direction is she going to step in the pool? She made herself vulnerable, took a step forward, by revealing her love of Italian food. What I did amounts to stomping on her big toe with the heel of a heavy work boot. Of course, she's going to step back! And, if I do something similar enough times, she's going to call an Uber to come get her and take her home.

A similar situation arose on my first date with my wife, Joanna. This was back in 1982, so let me set the scene a little for context.

I grew up a little way outside a West Texas town. I was in the FFA[1] in high school in which I won a couple of awards judging poultry (you heard me correctly), raising and showing pigs in the county fair, growing wheat and hay, and so on, you get the picture. At that point in my life, my taste in music was pretty much choked down to only liking classic rock and country. Also, being even more insecure about my manhood than I am now, I considered listening to pop music to be the part of the developmental stage that came right after *Barney* and *Sesame Street* songs. In 1982, a group from Australia called "Air Supply" was all the *pop* rage. On our first date, I asked Joanna what kind of music she liked. She said, "I love Air Supply." I couldn't imagine a worse answer. It took everything I had to keep my face from contorting into something that looked like I had just breathed in the fresh aroma of vomit while someone dragged their fingernails down a chalkboard. But the taste for such music was not a deal breaker for me. So, my reply was, "Hey, I heard Air Supply is doing a concert here next month. You wanna go?"

Was my answer a lie? Was I being less than forthcoming? No, I didn't say that I, too, liked *Air Supply*. I was simply trying my hardest to make her feel accepted by me. On top of that, I was already picturing myself with her at that concert, smiling, singing along, and having a great time. Because I liked Air Supply? No, because I would be with Joanna, doing what she liked.

Fast forward to 1987. Joanna and I have now been married for over two years, and things aren't going so well between us at this point. In fact, I'm beginning to think I married the wrong person, that I got married for the wrong reasons, that I'm not in love anymore, and that I don't like her anymore. (About five years later, she told me that she had been having all those same thoughts and feelings at that same time.)

So, we're riding in the car together and an Air Supply song comes on the radio. Simultaneously, I reach for the *change-the-station* knob as she reaches for the *turn-it-up* knob. An argument/power struggle ensues, and

---

[1] **Future Farmers of America**

I mention something to her about how terrible and cheesy this music is. And I'm wondering why my marriage is struggling!?![2]

You see, the shallow end is where we learn how the other person deals with things about us that are difficult for them to accept. Even if two people have the same beliefs, opinions, tastes, and preferences, ninety-nine percent of the time, there will still be differences one percent of the time. How they handle those differences is far more important than having similarities. If they don't handle the differences well, those differences will become what defines the relationship and begins to erode the intimacy and pleasant thoughts toward each other.

Back to acceptance. Remember, acceptance is at the core of why we look for a mate in the first place. But it is also at the core of what keeps the relationship growing and thriving for a lifetime. Without acceptance, everything else falls apart: communication, sex, intimacy, connectedness, trust, and so on. Internet dating services are based on the idea of compatibility. In and of itself, a certain degree of compatibility is important, but it is not the key. Because, no matter how compatible a couple seems to be, there will always be differences between the two that are difficult to accept.

About once a month, I conduct a three-day intensive workshop for struggling and failing marriages. Over the past fourteen years, I have conducted more than one hundred and twenty such workshops. One of the sessions of the workshop is about understanding and appreciating personality differences. We use one of the best-known personality assessments, the *DISC*, as a tool for looking at these personality differences. As Internet dating sites have become more and more mainstream, we have noticed a rise in the number of couples who score the same or similarly on this assessment. Almost every time this happens, one of the spouses will bring it to our attention. When they do, I love to ask the question, "Where did you two meet?" Because the answer is almost always, "On an Internet dating site." At which point I find great satisfaction in having

---

[2] **Joanna ended up going to the Air Supply concert with a guy named Mark. But that's a whole other story.**

a present and tangible example of how compatibility is not central to a successful marriage.

"You met on a sophisticated dating website that had you take a personality assessment, answer a bunch of questions about what you like and dislike, and then throw in a picture or two of yourself at your best," I will say. "This matched you up with someone who was considered compatible with yourself. You saw the pictures of them and probably had some instant sensual attraction. So, you read further and found out that they vote like you and enjoy the same music, food, and extracurricular activities as yourself and, low and behold, they seemed to have a similar personality to you. You just saved yourself a ton of money, energy, and time. You get to jump right in to the deep end together. So, you did! It felt so crazy-right from the get-go. You fell madly in love and each of you just knew you had found your soul mate. You got married six months later and now, five years after that, you can barely stand each other. What went wrong? You bought in to the idea that compatibility is the key."

Well, compatibility *is* important. Of course, if one of you is a bible-toting evangelical Christian and the other is a devout Muslim, you're going to have some major struggles! (By the way, I have worked with a couple of that precise mix. We'll get to them later.)

Please don't hear me saying that all Internet dating sites are bad. *Some* are extremely destructive. Heck, if I were thrown back into the dating scene because something happened to my wife, there are two or three dating sites that I would consider using, to help narrow down my search. But I would still make sure that any first dates would start at the shallow end of the pool.

Occasionally I will have someone bring up the idea of being equally yoked, a New Testament Scripture reference to choosing a spouse that is like-minded, more specifically, one that also follows the teachings of Jesus. A yoke is a device that joins two animals together and then is hitched to the plow that they are supposed to pull. The concept here is not that the two animals are similar. It's that they are pulling in the same direction. A two-thousand-pound bull that is yoked to his clone could be unequally yoked if the two animals are trying to pull in opposite directions. But, a two-hundred-pound donkey could be equally yoked to a two-thousand-pound bull if they are pulling in the same direction.

Joanna and I are very different in almost every sense of the term. She's of Mexican descent with black hair and brown skin. I'm of German and Swedish descent, and our wedding portrait looks like a snowball-headed kid standing next to Miss Latina USA. She's off-the-charts extraverted. I'm on the introverted side of the spectrum. Personality assessments have us as pretty much polar opposites. Heck, we've been married through nine Presidential Elections and have only voted for the same party two of those times. That alone would have been a deal breaker on the first speed date, and there's no way a dating site algorithm would have let us find each other. But after three and a half decades together, I can't imagine how boring and unfulfilling life would be without her.

So, in the shallow end of the pool, we take turns being vulnerable with each other. If our vulnerability is accepted, we feel a little safer and we take steps toward the deep end... deeper vulnerability. If our vulnerability is rejected, we step back to regain trust. Even people who have been married twenty or more years will have to come back to the shallow end, regularly, to feel safe and accepted enough to venture deeper. The couples I work with who are really struggling are almost always attempting to solve all their issues in the deep end, like two people trying to use each other as a floatation device, clawing and gasping to just be able to breathe. My first job is to lead them back to the shallow end. This usually seems counterintuitive to them at first. They believe that they must resolve the really big issues before they can deal with the lesser ones. However, neither one is going to feel safe enough to swim in the deep waters with the other until they have established trust in the shallow water.

Limerence:
The Science of Falling
in Love

Limerence:
The Science of Falling
in Love

So now we have this couple who have been successfully working their way toward the deep end. As they share more and more about themselves and, in turn, continue to show acceptance for what the other one shares, they each feel more and more accepted by the other. This feels incredible! It gets right at the core of our basic desire—to be accepted. It's the best feeling in the world. I accept you and, most importantly, you accept me. I feel so alive, so full of excitement and hope and energy! I think I'm in love! No, I *know* I'm in love! I know because you could tell me that the IRS is auditing me tomorrow and the only reason it would bother me is because it will mean time not spent with you. No biggie. We'll just do the audit together!

It is my personal observation that people who have been treated with the *least* amount of acceptance, in their past, fall in love quicker and easier than those who have been treated with more acceptance. The more you are used to not being accepted, the easier it is to see *unacceptance* as something to expect. So, a person who is only shown acceptance fifty percent of the time, with someone they are dating, might still believe they are being accepted if the last person they dated only showed them acceptance thirty percent of the time. This might sound like a good thing at first glance. It might look like they have thicker skin. But, once the limerence wears away, the rose-colored glasses come off and these people are often the ones whose relationships last the least amount of time. The easier it is to "fall in love," the easier it is to "fall out of love."

This feeling called "limerence," I will strongly argue, is the most sought-after feeling in the world. And once it's there, it becomes the most powerful physical phenomenon in the world. It's the single greatest source for movies, books, songs, poems, wardrobes, and, most importantly, haircuts. It's like a drug that will have you give up your job and family just to keep it. It is truly like cocaine or methamphetamines, more than you might imagine.

During this phase of the relationship, what most people call "in love," the brain isn't doing what it normally does. In fact, dopamine and nor-epinephrine levels are higher than normal, and serotonin levels are lower than normal.[1] As dopamine is being passed around in your brain at a higher rate, you are more motivated to do what it is that you're doing. Also, you have more desire for the object of what you're doing. When norepinephrine is increased, you have more energy and excitement. Norepinephrine actually makes you fart less when you are on an exciting date. What a great neurotransmitter!

Serotonin, on the other hand, drops during this phase. Serotonin functions to stabilize our mood. It also functions as an inhibitor. I like to call it the "Jiminy Cricket" neurotransmitter. If you remember the movie *Pinocchio*, you may recall that Jiminy Cricket rode around on Pinocchio's shoulder, trying to help him think before he did something stupid. He was Pinocchio's conscience. Well, when serotonin levels in our brain drop low, it's like thumping Jiminy off our shoulder. So, when someone is "madly in love," this chemical concoction that's floating around in his brain is doing the same thing as cocaine or meth. There's actually a scientific term for it: *limerence.*

---

[1] **The Harvard Mahoney Neuroscience Institute Letter, 2019**

The term "limerence" has been around for over fifty years. Over the past several decades, limerence has increasingly become one of the hottest fields of research in the behavioral and mental health sciences. My last Google of the term came up with almost a million results. To put that in perspective, I also Googled Fritz Haber and only came up with about half that many. Haven't heard of Fritz Haber either? He's the guy that basically saved half of the world from starving by inventing the process for making modern fertilizer. He also invented mustard gas and the gas used to kill millions in the gas chambers of the Holocaust. I mention this because most people have never heard of either limerence or Fritz Haber. But, that doesn't mean that they aren't extremely significant. In fact, so much of what we think we know comes from what our culture tells us rather than the facts. As the popular Simon and Garfunkel song "The Boxer" suggests, we tend to hear only what we want to hear and overlook everything else. I believe the reason that most people haven't heard of limerence is because they don't want to. Why don't they want to know about it? What's wrong with just keeping the good ole term "in love?"

Buckle up. The roller coaster of love is about to get even crazier.

Back in the 1960s, when people first began using actual science to study the universal phenomenon of falling in love, one of the leading researchers was a psychologist, Dr. Dorothy Tennov. As Tennov delved deeper and deeper, interviewing thousands of people who were experiencing this phenomenon, she began to realize that the term "love" was not an adequate term. So, she coined the term "limerence." Over the past thirteen years, I have read every research article I can find on the subject. Along with my experience of personally working with thousands of couples, here are some fascinating things I have learned so far.

No two people experience limerence in exactly the same way. Some go through it quicker than others. Some experience the feelings more intensely than others. Some experience limerence, but the other person (limerent object) does not. And then there's all the other things that make limerence a unique experience to each person, such as personality, upbringing, and prior experiences. So, at the risk of over-generalizing, here are a couple of "textbook" examples of people in limerence:

The Coworker

You've worked with him for three years. He is the definition of responsible: always on time or early, always finishes each job ahead of schedule or better than required, never takes a sick day, and so on. Then, one day, he begins to have a relationship with the woman down the hall. A few months go by and now he's used up all his sick leave and often gets back from lunch late. Everyone knows it has something to do with her.

The Seventeen-Year-Old Daughter

She's what most parents want in a daughter. She makes good grades. She makes good choices. She's compliant with her teachers and gets along well with her parents. Then she starts to date this guy that her dad does not approve of. Finally, he confronts her.

Dad: "I don't think this guy is good for you."

Daughter: "That's because you don't know him. If you knew him like I do, you'd think he's wonderful!"

Dad: "Well, it's true that I don't know him as well as you, but I do know that he has been arrested twice for dealing drugs."

Daughter: "Well, duh! That's because he's trying to earn money for college!"

When people are in limerence, they are not their normal selves.

Let's first understand one of the most important things to know about limerence: it does *not* last.

That's right, limerence goes away 100% of the time. And I'm not talking about death, although that is one way to end it. On average, limerence lasts about a year, more specifically, six to eighteen months. In a small percentage of cases, it lasts up to three years, and in some very rare cases, it can last up to five years. So, what's the secret to making it last longer? Well, it's very simple:

Stay away from the person you are in limerence with!

Because, you see, the greatest single factor that determines how long limerence lasts is how much the relationship is exposed to "real life." To help understand why this is, let's first start with a helpful definition:

Limerence: the illusion of complete acceptance

The more you do "real life" with someone, the more you discover things about him or her that you don't accept and, of course, the more they discover about you that *they* don't accept. As you discover more and more about each other that is not acceptable, the more the illusion of complete acceptance is diminished. Here's a textbook example of limerence that lasts for three years:

The Office Affair

He lives in Los Angeles and has been married for eight years with two children. She lives in New York, has been married for seven years, and has three children. Neither one would say that they have a bad marriage. Both would report being committed to their marriage, but both are discovering that their marriages aren't as fulfilling and exciting as they were expecting. Both work for a company that is based in Denver. About once a month, the company flies them both to Denver for a few days because they are both part of the same team that is working on a mutual project. After this goes on for a few months, they begin to get to know each other a little more, and each feels that the relationship is safe because neither has any particular *sensual* attraction to the other (i.e., physical attraction). Also, they each see the relationship as relatively safe because they are just coworkers, nothing more.

At first, their discussions are only work-related but, nonetheless, interesting and exciting, because their work is something they are both really in to and it's about the things that interest both of them. One day when the work day is winding down, they agree to finish talking shop over a drink in the hotel bar, the hotel they are both staying in because it's where the company pays for them to stay. Without realizing it, they have both now taken a step into the shallow end. They don't realize it because they weren't sensually attracted to each other. But, there was a cognitive attraction because they are both really into this common big part of their lives—their project. During the work day, what they hear from each other is what the rest of the team hears. But now, with just the two of them, they begin to share some ideas, about the project, that they are not sure the rest of the team will accept. So, they are making themselves vulnerable to each other. As they show each other acceptance for their respective ideas, they begin to wade deeper into the pool together and are now up to their waists (no pun intended). After a while the conversation turns from work to matters that are a little more personal. They begin to ask each other about their homelife.

"Tell me about your wife," she says.

"Oh, she's a great lady and a good mom," he replies. "What about you? What's your marriage like?"

"Oh, he's a good man as well. I love him but I have to admit, marriage is hard sometimes. It's definitely not what I thought it was going to be."

"I totally get that. I guess marriage is just hard work," he says.

"But I don't believe it has to be. I think some people just marry the wrong person," she says. "Do you think you married the right person?"

"Sometimes I wonder," he replies.

"Me too," she agrees.

They then share this awkward but exciting moment of silence. They have both taken some bold steps into deeper vulnerability, and both felt understood and accepted. He then declares that he needs to head back to his room and answer some emails. She agrees that she needs to do the same. Close call!

The next night after work, with nothing else they have to do, he asks if she wants to continue last night's conversation at the hotel restaurant. He uses the seemingly innocent "we gotta eat something" excuse. That night the conversation deepens, and they find themselves beginning to now be sensually attracted to each other. After a few months of this, the relationship becomes a full-blown extramarital affair. They are now in crazy limerence. Twenty-seven days of the month are spent doing "real life" back at home with all the domestic hassles, bills to pay, parenting duties, and a marriage that has become stagnant. Three days out of the month, all that stuff is a thousand miles away. Their food, lodging, and transportation are all taken care of by the company. The only decisions they have to make together are the ones they are both excited about and agree on—their work project.

So, a year goes by. Since they are only with each other three days out of the month, they have been experiencing limerence at less than one-tenth the rate of a couple who sees each other on a daily basis and must work through everyday matters together. Because this limerence has lasted so long, they are even more convinced that they are each other's *true love*. So, they divorce their spouses, move to Denver, and buy a house together.

A few weeks after they move in together, he notices that she hasn't offered to cook dinner even once, something his ex-wife did almost every night. When she asks him to rub her feet, something her ex-husband did for her almost every night, he exclaims that he is not into foot rubbing. Then they begin to notice other things they would like to change about each other: She rolls her eyes at him when she doesn't agree with how he thinks he should deal with his children; he interrupts her when she begins to explain a viewpoint of hers that he doesn't agree with; she thinks the toilet paper roll should be mounted to the dispenser so that it feeds from the top; and he thinks toilet paper should feed from the bottom because it's easier for him to grab and tear that way. As they discover these things they don't like about each other, they begin to recognize, more and more, that they do *not* accept everything about each other. So, the limerence begins to fade. Another two years go by and not only has the limerence faded, but their efforts to change what they don't like about each other have left the other feeling totally unaccepted, and things are now worse than they were with their former spouses.

So why have most people never heard of limerence, even though there is so much written about it and so much research, for more than fifty years now? Here's one big reason: most of us don't *want* to know about it! We all like the term "in love" because it implies something pure and lasting… something that was destined to be. We want to believe that, whenever we are in it, and whoever we are in it with, it's ultimately good. And, if it goes away with one person and comes back with someone else, well, then what we had with that previous person wasn't true love and what we have now, since it feels so strong, must be the real, true love, making it justifiable, no matter who it is with.

I have worked with literally hundreds of couples in which one of the spouses is in limerence with someone else. The reasons I hear, for justifying the affair, are often so crazy that only someone in limerence would believe them. For example, I have worked with many who were involved in an extramarital affair with someone in their church. Often, they are very involved with their church, and several have even been ministers or pastors of that church. They will say things like, "I know that this is a good thing and that it was meant to be because we are on the worship team together."

But another reason we don't want to know about limerence is because it implies much more self-responsibility than we want to take on. We want to believe that there is someone out there who, if we find them, will fully accept us. And, if that's the case, we don't have to grow. In other words, we don't have to get better at loving. We can stay in our state of arrested development and things will be great. But loving people doesn't come naturally. We aren't born lovers. We are born takers. We come out of the womb with only the desire to be served and taken care of. We are not thinking of others' wants and needs, only our own. When is the last time you saw a three-year old sincerely ask someone, "what can I do to help?" Love is not something we *feel*, it's something we *do*. Love is a learned, practiced discipline, as cold as that may seem to our romantic sensibilities.

A lot of people get hung up on the idea of love being action instead of feeling. Many pass that notion off as just some sort of ancient religious sentiment to help us stay married or be nicer people. But, as a psychologist, I can tell you that it is also a scientific truth. When you love someone, you can feel any and every emotion there is: sadness, joy, anger, excitement, depression, grief, warmth, anxiety, and so on.

Love is also not a thought or way of thinking. Anyone, who has been married for more than a few days, can tell you that they have had some pretty negative thoughts about, and toward, their spouse. If you've been married more than a few years, you've likely had a brief thought or two about choking your spouse. But, in some of those moments, you instead decided to do something loving. In fact, those are the moments when you are being the most loving. It takes little or no love to be nice to someone when they are being nice to you. Love is most defined in those moments when our actions are counter to our unpleasant feelings. Limerence is a way of thinking and a powerful set of feelings. Limerence is not a way of doing. Therefore, limerence is not love.

But, limerence is great when it is appropriate! So, don't hear me saying that limerence is a bad thing. Just because it's not, in and of itself, love, doesn't mean that it's a bad thing. Fresh fruit, most would agree, is a good thing... a gift from God. But that doesn't make it love. One reason I state this is because, as I was first learning about limerence, I started to get really frustrated because it seemed like one big cruel joke that nature plays on us. We have these super-intense and pleasant feelings with someone, so we decide to get married, and then, shortly thereafter, the feelings go away, and we wake up one day wondering what happened to that person we had fallen in love with.

As a sidenote to make this point, women typically experience a higher sex drive than normal, and men are typically more thoughtful and helpful during limerence. It reminds me of a joke I once heard that went something like this:

Question: How do you get a woman to stop having sex with you?
Answer: Marry her.

Now as awful and sexist as that joke is, you've probably heard similar jokes and statements made about men as well that support what everyone, who has been married for more than a few years, seems to instinctively know—something changes from when you first "fall in love" to a year or two later. Why? Why can't the limerence last for life? Why this big trick of nature? Or, if you are a person of faith, why does God do this to us? These are important questions! Questions that had me very frustrated as I was beginning to learn about the limerence phenomenon. But then I began to discover some things that make so much sense. So, let's look at those things.

The Stuff of Love Songs

Have you ever noticed that there are two basic themes to all love songs?

Theme A: This is the best feeling in the world.

This theme gives us such songs as "The Air That I Breathe" and "I Can't Live Without You."

Theme B: How do I get that feeling back.

This theme gives us such songs as "You've Lost That Loving Feeling" and "Trying to Get the Feeling Again."

Now if you look at the timeline of the average limerence experience, which is roughly twelve months, we can think of that timeline as a bell curve.

The Limerence Phase

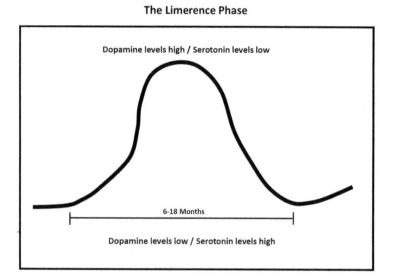

Dopamine levels high / Serotonin levels low

6-18 Months

Dopamine levels low / Serotonin levels high

At the beginning of the curve, as it is moving upward, dopamine and norepinephrine levels are increasing as serotonin levels are dropping.

Limerence is increasing. Said another way, the illusion of full acceptance is increasing. The other side of the curve is where neurotransmitters are going back to their normal state. Limerence is now decreasing. The illusion of full acceptance is going away. So, the left side of the graph, where limerence is increasing, is love song theme A: This is the best feeling in the world. When we are in this state, nothing else really seems to matter, only being with that other person. I have dealt with numerous couples in which one spouse is involved in an extramarital affair and has suddenly become disinterested in the children... often neglectful. You also see more severe versions of this almost daily in the news, for example, the person who is involved with someone who is not the other parent of their child. So, the child is neglected, abandoned, and, yes, sometimes, even murdered!

The right side of the curve, where limerence is fading, is love song theme B: How do I get the feeling back. This is where the neurotransmitters are returning to their normal state, where we begin to return to a more rational and responsible state. Remember, the two stages together, theme A and theme B, last about twelve months. What happens in these twelve months? A lot of sex! What tends to happen when there's a lot of sex going on? Babies!

It should be noted that many couples are committed to saving sex until the wedding night. There are many good reasons for doing so. The majority of reputable research shows that people who have had no other sexual partner other than their spouse have greater sexual satisfaction with their spouses, are less likely to divorce, are less likely to have sex outside the marriage, and have higher levels of trust with their spouse.[2] That being said, most of those do not abstain from intercourse with each other until their honeymoon. They're still having premarital sex with each other. Furthermore, they are often doing so without any form of

---

[2] **Notre Dame Journal of Law, Ethics & Public Policy**
Volume 18 Issue 1Symposium on Marriage and the Law Article 2
1-1-2012 Saying Yes Before Saying I Do: Premarital Sex and Cohabitation as a Piece of the Divorce Puzzle, Helen M. Alvare

birth control because they are not "planning" on having sex. Rather, they are planning on saving themselves for each other on their wedding night. So, whether people are just in uncommitted limerence, engaged, or married and still in limerence, this is where most of the couples' first-borns are conceived. What happens if the limerence doesn't go away before the child is born? At best, the child is going to experience severe diaper rash from spending hours in a dirty diaper because mom and dad are too wrapped up in each other to notice... at best. In other words, if limerence doesn't go away, far fewer babies survive. And the ones that do will likely have abandonment and neglect issues or worse. So, the fading of limerence is nature's way of helping us to get past the idea that all we need is each other so that we can focus some of our time, energy, and resources on the well-being of the child. Limerence lasts about a year. Pregnancies last about nine months. Perfect timing! Also, people in limerence don't care as much about domestic responsibilities. It needs to go away so that we can refocus some of our energy on keeping up with other things such as our job or cleaning the dishes that are piling up and attracting roaches.

But that only explains the right side of the curve. Why does there need to be a curve at all? Wouldn't it be better if there was no limerence at all so that we don't get "tricked" into putting on the rose-colored glasses of believing we are fully accepted and that we fully accept the other? Wouldn't it be better if we really knew what we were getting into before we decide to marry? It seems like we would be way better off if there was no limerence and we just took the time and effort to really get to know someone before we decided to even date them, much less get married and start a family together!

One answer to this is, in my mind, straightforward: we definitely should get to know someone well before we start dating them. We don't choose who we will have limerence with. We only choose who to test out the pool with. There is no good reason to even step into a pool with someone you know would not be a good mate, much less a good parent.

The other part of the answer is this: we are all told that marriage is not easy and that it's hard work. You have to make sacrifices. You must put *me* aside for the sake of *us*. Also, the data has been overwhelmingly clear since the data began being collected, over sixty years ago[3]: people raised by parents who are married to each other are better off than people who aren't raised with both parents still married to each other. So, marriage isn't all rainbows and unicorns, but we have even fewer rainbows and unicorns without it.

So, imagine that everyone has a *YouTube* video of what your life would be if the two of you were married to each other. The video shows all the good stuff you go through together, but it also shows all the bad: arguments, sacrifices, struggles, times when you felt abandoned, and times you felt betrayed, all the stuff that *every* marriage goes through because every marriage is made up of two human beings who have issues and spend more time thinking of their own needs and desires than others. If this were the case, if we could see into that possible future, it's doubtful that any of us would get married. So, without limerence to "trick" us into becoming a committed spouse and parent, children wouldn't have the hope of a healthy family. And, just as important, we wouldn't take the step of commitment to marriage, which is the main crucible of learning how to truly love. Limerence jump-starts lifelong love. But limerence, in and of itself, is not love.

Now this may be sounding like marriage, and children for that matter, is not going to lead to a happy life. And, in fact, many in our culture are saying that marriage is a concept that is out of date and impractical. As we move along, those ideas will be shown to be false, so hang in there. In fact, most studies on happiness and marriage show that married people are, overall, happier than unmarried people.[4] This becomes more and more evident when couples get past that classic "seven-year itch."

---

[3] **US Census Bureau, 2010, 2000, 1990, 1980, 1970, 1960**

[4] **Grover, S. S., Helliwell, J. F., How's Life At Home? New Evidence on Marriage and the Setpoint for Happiness, Journal of Happiness Studies, December, 2017**

[5]For example, one study found that couples who have been married for at least thirty-five years have, on average, higher levels of dopamine and norepinephrine and lower levels of serotonin. When you've been through a lot of real life with someone, the good and the bad, but wake up and roll over, for the twelve thousandth time, and see that same person lying beside you, still choosing you over everyone else, the *illusion* of acceptance begins to be the *reality* of acceptance.

---

[5] In 2002, there was an extensive study completed by a team of highly respected researchers, led by University of Chicago Sociologist Linda Waite.* The team gave an assessment to 5,232 married adults to determine the level of satisfaction each had with their marriage. Five years later they gave each person the same assessment. Of those who first reported being the most unhappy in their marriage yet remained married to that same person, five years later, eighty percent now reported being happily married! It is apparent that something changed. But, just as important as the change that occurred, something had to be in place to keep them engaged in the marriage long enough for that change to occur. That thing that kept them engaged? Something that has seemed to take on a different meaning with each passing generation. Something called "commitment." We will get to that soon enough.

INTIMACY: THE COMPLEX SIMPLICITY

Intimacy: The Complex Simplicity

E veryone desperately craves intimacy because it's what most makes us feel accepted, the very core of what motivates us. However, everyone also greatly *fears* intimacy because it requires that we be vulnerable. And, when we are vulnerable, it's easier to get hurt.

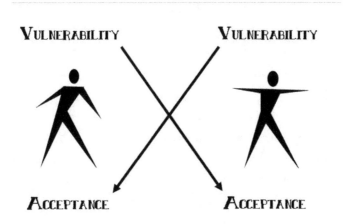

The picture above illustrates what intimacy is. In simple terms, it's two or more people being vulnerable with each other and those same people accepting the vulnerability that the other(s) is revealing. Most people today use the terms "sex" and "intimacy" interchangeably, but people can have sex without it being intimate, and intimacy can happen without having sex. Good, healthy intimacy can happen between practically any two people: mother and son, father and daughter, siblings, close friends, and so on. If two people are sharing thoughts with each other that they don't normally share with the public and they both are accepting what the other is sharing, they are experiencing intimacy. One reason intimacy may have become more and more associated with only sex is because many seem to be finding it more and more difficult to be vulnerable with thoughts and feelings that are more profound and guarded. But intimate sex, like intimate conversation, still follows this simple pattern of two people being vulnerable and each accepting the vulnerability of the other.

The vulnerability of sex is obvious. When you take off all your clothes, in front of someone, they are literally seeing parts of you that the world doesn't get to see. And, of course, they are doing the same. But, suppose I had a big, hairy mole on my rear end that was in the shape of Oklahoma. And, the first time I get naked in front of my wife, she can now see it. She might say something like, "Oh, that's so cute! It reminds me of the Ozarks in the Fall!" Of course, with a loving and sincere delivery, that would show me acceptance. However, if instead she said, "Ewww! That thing looks like a big hairy Oklahoma," well, the intimacy has been interrupted. (By the way, so you don't get too distracted here, it's actually shaped like Australia.)

Sex is so loaded with potential land mines that it can be very scary for a lot of people. Likewise, intimate conversation can be very scary for people who have been really hurt by revealing their thoughts and ideas. Although there are other ways to achieve intimacy, sex and conversation are the two most common avenues. On top of that, most people prefer one over the other. This is usually because the preferred method of intimacy is the one for which they have the least amount of fear of getting hurt. You may be thinking that it's usually the men who prefer sex and the women who prefer conversation. While that is more typical, it is very often the opposite. There are many women who prefer sex, and there are many men who prefer conversation. Either way, what is almost always the case is that they marry someone who prefers a different method, of achieving intimacy, from themselves.

It's not like we go around asking potential dates which one they prefer. There's no sign hanging around our neck to indicate which one we prefer. I've worked with literally thousands of couples. In counseling with them, and often in smaller group workshops, I will ask which form of intimacy they prefer. In all but two of the cases, each person preferred the one that their spouse *didn't* prefer. I'm pretty sure that one of those exceptions was just a husband who was trying to score brownie points with his wife.

What's going on here? How does this happen? Could it be that we are wired to seek out a mate that is so fundamentally different from ourselves? How would this serve us? It seems that it would only make lifelong love even more difficult to achieve than it is. It certainly doesn't serve to make it any easier! Yet, it is overwhelmingly the case that most of us instinctively choose a mate who prefers to achieve intimacy in the manner that we do *not* prefer. What if pushing ourselves out of our own comfort zone, and more into the comfort zone of our spouse, makes us more complete?

In the Bible, at the very beginning, it states:

So God created mankind in God's own image. In the image of God, God created them; male and female God created them.

If this is true, that would mean that even if I were perfect, I would only be half of the image of God. Maybe, the more I learn to love in the way that is least comfortable to me, the more I am becoming a complete image. Something to think about!

All marriages have conflict. We will have conflict with anyone we spend a significant amount of time with. Now, it's important to understand that conflict is neither good nor bad. It's what we *do* with conflict that can be good or bad. But conflict, in and of itself, simply means that there is a difference that doesn't match up. It could be a difference of opinion, a difference in taste, a difference of notion of what to do for the evening together; conflict is simply when the differences collide, and that will happen on almost a daily basis between any two people who are sharing a roof and domestic responsibilities. Conflict is only bad when it is not resolved for the good of both parties.

When two people are experiencing intimacy with each other and a conflict arises, it interrupts the intimacy. The interruption can last a lifetime if the conflict is not settled. Or, it can last less than a second or anywhere in between.

When a marriage starts out, there is usually a lot of intimacy going on, especially if both are still in limerence. He is pushing himself out of his comfort zone to do intimacy in her preferred way. And, she is pushing herself out of her comfort zone to do intimacy in his preferred way. But, along the way, sometimes it doesn't go so well. One night he laughs at a sound she makes while having sex. One day she mocks him for being too intense about one of his values. As these sorts of things begin to happen, they each begin to trust each other a little less in the deep end. At the same time, they both desperately crave being in the deep end together because that is where the best things they've experienced together have happened. So, they continue to try to work these things out from that deep end. When conversation goes badly, but they can't seem to resolve it together, the one who prefers sex as a means of intimacy tries to solve it by dropping the matter and just having sex. This is what a lot of people refer to as "makeup sex." But the argument couldn't be resolved, so the moment is not truly intimate. They want to be intimate again but don't know how to resolve the conversational conflict, so they try to go around the conflict back to intimacy, through sex. But something about it doesn't feel as intimate as before because the conflict wasn't resolved. The same happens with the sexual conflict. Something doesn't go so well in bed, the sexual interaction comes to a halt, and, later, they try to resolve it through conversation. Over time, both the sex and the conversations become less and less because neither feels like they are safe in the others' preferred arena of intimacy.

The solution to this vicious cycle is twofold:

1. Each must push him or herself even harder to initiate intimacy in the way the other prefers, *especially* if the other one isn't making an effort to get out of their comfort zone.
2. Each must invite the other to shallower waters when it comes to doing intimacy in the way the other least prefers.

Easier said than done, right? It's easier than you think if you go back to dating again.

DATE FOR LIFE

Date for Life

Once people get married, they often believe they are now finished with the dating phase of their relationship, so they quit doing the things that got them into limerence in the first place:

Being attractive
Being vulnerable
Being accepting

As I mentioned earlier, Joanna and I went through this phase in about years two and three of our marriage. That's when we didn't like each other anymore and our marriage was struggling. During that time, we lived about five hundred miles from both sets of parents, and Joanna was spending more and more evenings on the phone with her mom and dad. Some of those were, no doubt, tear-filled. One day I get a call from her dad saying that he wants to sign us up for a marriage seminar that was going to take place in another state. That was the last thing I wanted to do. I tried to come up with excuses, but he was not taking "no" for an answer. So, we went to our first marriage seminar.

To this day, I only remember two things that I learned from that seminar:

1. Good marriages don't just happen by marrying the right person.
2. Don't ever stop dating each other.

In other words, if you're going to have a good marriage, you're going to have to work at it. Some people have such a hard time with this concept. They want to believe that if it's real love, it will just come naturally and without effort. Where does that come from? What else in life follows the rule of "What's good for you will come naturally"?

Liking vegetables doesn't come naturally. Liking sugar does.

Liking exercise doesn't come naturally. Liking to sit and be entertained does.

Thinking about the well-being of others does not come naturally. Looking out for yourself does.

Those who never grow out of the mindset that love just naturally happens will never have close, meaningful relationships that last. Instead, they will move from mate to mate, leaving a wake of destruction that will fold itself back onto their own lives, not to mention the destruction to others.

But, even though a lot of people think that marriage is hard work, it is much easier than single life, if done well. What makes it seem like such hard work for many is that they are constantly climbing in and out of the deep end, just to be able to catch enough breath to jump back into that deep end to try to work things out. But, most of that work is only going to be accomplished in the shallow end, where both feel safe. Even the best marriages spend at least as much time in the shallow end as they do in the deep end. But they also spend more time in the deep end than people of bad marriages, because they are able to relax and enjoy the deep end more. They do this by continuing to date each other.

Back to that marriage seminar. As I mentioned, one of my big takeaways was to keep dating. So, Joanna and I started planning regular dates together, almost every week. But our dates weren't going so well. We were often arguing before we even got to the restaurant. On top of that, we were going broke because we were now "dating" so much. But, we kept at it because we had learned that you gotta keep dating. Over time, I began to resent date night. Not only was it usually a disaster, it was making it more and more difficult to pay our bills. So, what were we doing wrong?

One thing I had forgotten was that when we first started dating,

Joanna and I dated almost every day. But we were broke college students. We couldn't afford to do dinner and movie even once a week. That probably happened more like once a month. And, it was usually something like Taco Bell and the bargain theater that showed movies that had been out for half a year. Not to mention, we probably snuck in our own refreshments instead of spending twenty dollars on two sodas and a bucket of popcorn. But we dated several times a week. Sometimes that date was just a walk or a bike ride. Sometimes it was just sitting in her parents' living room. Sometimes it was a picnic. Sometimes it was just a two-hour talk on the phone. It's not a fancy dinner or exciting entertainment that qualifies something as a "date."[1] It's what you did on those dates:

Be attractive
Be vulnerable
Be accepting

It was early fall, 1982. A new men's foot fashion had just made its way into our little town. Me and my buddies called them "boat shoes." They also went by the terms "deck shoes," "Top-Sider's," and "Sperry's."

Joanna and I were at a restaurant called "O'Malley's" on what was probably our fifth or sixth date. As we sat there talking and eating, a guy walks by our table wearing a pair of these Sperry's. Now, in 1982 I had three basic sets of footwear: my work boots, my Sunday-go-to-meetin' boots, and my athletic shoes. Well, as this guy passed our table, I saw Joanna's eyes lock onto his shoes. Once he got around the corner, Joanna turned to me and, in a low voice, said, "You'd look good in a pair of those." What I felt, in that moment, was something akin to being told I had to

---

[1] This doesn't mean that we should be cheapskates. If you're investing more time and money into a hobby or buying things for yourself than you are on your relationship, you aren't going to have much intimacy. One of the things it took me about two decades to figure out is that Joanna feels a lot more loved by me when I plan a date out ahead of time. Even if I don't get all the details just the way she would prefer, investing time and money into making reservations at a nice restaurant of my choosing means a lot more to her than waiting until we get in the car and saying, "I'll happily let you choose where we go eat, as long as it's less than thirty dollars."

wear a tutu to school. I don't even remember if I replied because I didn't know how to say "Are you high?" without it coming across negatively. What I do know, however, is that the next day I'm at Target when I spot, on the endcap of one of the shoe aisles, a display of what looked like the same type of shoe that Joanna had been referring to the night before. I think they might have even been named "Target Siders." The price was way less than what you would have paid for a pair of "Top-Sider's." They had that extra lace running through eyelets around the ankle. They had that same white rubber sole. They resembled something made of leather. The only difference that I could detect was that they didn't have that little sailboat stamped on the heel. Oh, and one other minor detail, instead of being that classic buckskin-tan color, it appeared to be the case that they had been spray-painted in a glossy taupe. Again, a minor detail (in my mind).

A few days later, I show up at her door, ready for our seventh date, wearing my new Target Siders. Joanna noticed them right away because I kept looking down at the shoes, then back to her, then down at the shoes again, as I smiled with the satisfaction I had from knowing that I was impressing her *and* saving about fifty dollars. I could tell she was impressed because she could have won an Academy Award for how well she made me believe that she liked them. Years later she told me that she had never loved a pair of shoes more… or hated a pair of shoes more. She hated them because they were so ugly. She loved them because she knew that I had gone waaaay out of my comfort zone in attempt to be attractive to her.

Sometimes we get the idea that being attractive means looking like you're eighteen again. Well time and gravity take their toll on all of us. And remember that attraction doesn't just mean sensual. Cognitive and affective attractions are just as important. And, in fact, affective attraction tends to run much deeper. The mere effort to be attractive can be a pretty powerful attraction, in and of itself.

Five years into our marriage and we were going out on our weekly, miserable dates. Instead of being attractive, I was wearing what I felt comfortable in and what I thought was more representative of the real me. Before we married, I did my best to dress in what I thought was attractive to Joanna. Now, I was using date time to attempt to sway her to my point of view on issues and matters of life. Before we were married, I would ask about her and what she liked and disliked. Now, when her thoughts, tastes, and ideas were not in line with mine, I would ridicule her for having them. And, I couldn't understand why date night was going so horribly wrong.

Dates with your spouse should only be about getting to know each other more and accepting what you find out. Dating is the shallow end of the pool that is the foundation for building the trust and acceptance that are so crucial for making the deep end meaningful. Here are a few rules of thumb for successful "date time":

Don't try to solve anything between the two of you.
Don't bring up any issues that you know you disagree on.
Don't try to change your spouse's mind about anything.
Don't confront your spouse about anything.

We've even suggested couples have a sacred space in their house where none of these things are allowed. And, we recommend that there be regular, even daily, time in that space together. It could simply be a room that is understood by both of you as the safe place. It's the place that both of you understand as the shallow end. Nobody is going to hold me under here.

CONFLICT CREATES INTIMACY

CONFLICT
CREATES INTIMACY

If you think about it, conflict is a necessary ingredient for intimacy. Again, conflict doesn't mean argument or battle, it simply means difference that has not been resolved. It could even be argued that there is no intimacy *without* conflict. One reason for this is that intimacy requires at least two human beings who are interacting with each other. And, any two human beings who are regularly interacting with each other are going to have conflict. But another reason that intimacy requires conflict is because it is the conflict, itself, that is the necessary hurdle that must be overcome in order to have true intimacy.

When two people first start dating and begin the limerence process together, they will likely experience many intimate moments. And, it is likely that they will see those intimate moments as the result of something they have in common. To put it more plainly, they will believe that the intimate moment is the result of "sameness." But, if that was the case, then there must have been a difference (conflict) right before that moment. The common ground that they had reached, when they felt intimate, was the conflict (difference) being resolved. The scenario might have played out something like this:

Her: "What do you think about watching CSI after we eat?"

Him: "Oh, I can't stand those shows, it's always the same thing… somebody was sexually abused and then murdered by their seemingly innocent stepfather."

Her: "Well, what do you wanna watch then?

Him: "How about a Marvel or DC Comics movie?"

Her: "You mean a superhero movie? Where somebody has some unique superpower?"

Him: "Well… yeah."

Her: "And you think CSI is always the same story? How can you get more same story than a superhero movie?"

Him: "I also like old reruns from my childhood."

Her: "Ooooh, I love *Gilligan's Island*!"

Thirty minutes later while watching *Gilligan's Island* together…

Him: "This is so cool that I've finally found someone to watch *Gilligan's Island* with!"

Her: "I knew there was something special and different about you!"

So, you see, the intimacy was the result of their differences. When they found common ground, and a way to solve those differences, they experienced intimacy. Think of it in another way: You couldn't have intimacy with your clone (supposing you had a clone). If your clone always wanted to do the same thing as you, which he or she would naturally want to do because it's your clone, for crying out loud, that wouldn't feel special. The reason your clone wants to do those things has nothing to do with trying to please you or show you acceptance. The reason the clone wants to do those things is because that's what the clone wants to do, with or without you. Intimacy is the result of difference, not sameness.

Many couples, especially ones who have been married less than two years, experience times when they attempt to achieve intimacy without resolving the conflict that is interfering with it. They have a disagreement that turns into an argument. They both begin to feel angry, frustrated, and hurt by each other. They don't like those feelings, but they don't know how to resolve the conflict. So, they decide to just have sex, hoping for instant intimacy. This is often referred to as "makeup sex," which can be a good thing if the conflict is first resolved. But when it isn't, the sex is not as intimate, and, over time, as this begins to be the norm in situations where the conflict is not resolved, one or the other begins to feel used and sex begins to feel more and more "cheap." The same can happen with intimate conversation. When a conflict is unresolved but both are feeling a growing frustration and hurt, they may try to just change the subject, hoping to get back to intimacy through a subject that they agree on. But the conflict is left unresolved, and one or both begins to feel like conversations between the two are becoming more and more about sweeping aside thoughts and feelings, as if their own beliefs and values don't matter enough to be heard. Before long, both sex and conversation begin to diminish as both feel increasingly betrayed by the other for seeming to deny them from the form of intimacy that they are desiring. One is withholding sex because the other is withholding conversation because the one is withholding sex because the other is withholding conversation because....

I recently had a couple tell me that this was their situation. They asked me how to break the cycle.

First off, I told them, you gotta stop withholding what the other person wants, even if they seem unwilling to stop withholding what you want. Second, you must start resolving your conflicts. And, you're going to have to start in the shallow end. The two of you are attempting to resolve all your conflicts in the deep end where you both feel so unaccepted by each other that you're essentially clawing to keep your head above water by using each other as a life preserver. Resolving conflict. Easier said than done, right? In a few chapters, we will look at a way to resolve it quickly in almost every situation. But first let's spend some time addressing some very common but destructive mindsets.

THE UNBEARABLE
BURDEN

THE UNBEARABLE BURDEN

G et out a pen or pencil.
Yes, I mean now.

Take a moment to look at the list below and circle every word that you think represents a necessary ingredient for a good marriage. (If you are reading this on an electronic device such as your smartphone or kindle, I recommend not writing on the screen. Instead, get out a sheet of paper and write down any of the words that you consider a necessary ingredient for a good marriage.)

love	honor	trust	affection
attraction	compassion	intimacy	honesty
teamwork	acceptance	passion	sex
kindness	faithfulness	consideration	tenderness
hope	gentleness	adventure	warmth
shared goals	respect	compromise	good communication
friendship	forgiveness	understanding	commitment
shared purpose	vulnerability	openness	fun
healthy boundaries	understanding	joy	patience
peace	fidelity	self-control	passion

How many did you circle? In other words, how many of these things are important and/or necessary ingredients to a good marriage? There are fifty terms. I'm sure you could come up with at least one or two more that you think are important. But the question is: how many of these terms represent something that you believe is important for a good marriage?

I think they all are, all fifty of them, plus some more. But what about you? Would you say that at least forty of them are necessary for a good marriage? How about thirty? Twenty? Let's just say, for argument's sake, that you only believe that three of them are important for a good marriage. As long as two people are consistently doing three of these things, they will have a good marriage. My question would be: who consistently does any three of these things? Who is always trustworthy? Who is always 100% committed? Who is always loving? Who is always compassionate, self-controlled, kind, and so on? I think we can all agree that the answer is...

Nobody.

Even on my best days, I fall short of totally being even three things that it takes to be a good spouse.

This begs the question: who can have a good marriage?

I don't know about you, but I have seen lots of good marriages that are made up of two people who are consistently less than an ideal spouse. Now that I think about it, all the good marriages, I know of, are made up of two individuals who are often selfish, uncompassionate, unreasonable, irritable, frustrating, and so on.

However, when a marriage is not going well, my experience is that at least one of the two spouses is focused on all the things that the other person is *not* doing perfectly. They are wasting their time and energy trying to get the other to be better at being a spouse, believing that the marriage will be better if the other person would simply *behave* better. Once someone has bought into that mindset, the marriage *cannot* get better, even if the other person becomes almost perfect in consistently doing and being all those things. The marriage *cannot* get better for the person in this mindset, because this mindset requires the other person to be ideal, in order to be happy in the marriage.

I love backpacking. I love the outdoors and spending time in natural settings. But what I love most about backpacking is the idea that, at least for a short time, I can survive and even thrive with only the things I can carry on my back. There's something very satisfying to me when I'm out in the wilderness for a few days and I realize that so much of what I think I need in this life I don't really need. Even though most of us have never done rigorous "survival" stuff like a weeklong backpacking trip, miles from electricity, running water, and permanent shelter, I think most of us have some of the "backpacker" spirit in us. We like to fantasize that if our backs were up against the wall, we would have what it takes to survive. I think this notion has a lot to do with why dystopian movies and zombie apocalypse TV shows are so popular—we like to imagine ourselves not needing all those things that we so often tell ourselves we need, that we are capable enough to function in a "less than" environment. Again, this goes back to acceptance. If I can't be useful to others without some of the things I do have, how would I really matter to the group if I had more? What would matter would not really be about me, only the material things I have.

Well, when Joanna and I started talking about getting married, I began to think of our marriage as a lifelong backpacking trip together. We each had our proverbial backpack that was full of the things that we believed were essential to survive and even thrive in this world, many of the things on the list above. Although we both had some of the same things, we also had some things in our own backpack that the other person didn't believe was important enough to be burdened with carrying for the rest of her or his life. For example, one of the things that were in my backpack was what I will call *frequent-and-exciting-sexual-intimacy.* Although Joanna sees an importance in sexual intimacy in marriage, she wouldn't have had this same item in her backpack. She might have had an item called *meaningful-sexual-intimacy-on-special-occasions.* On the other hand, Joanna had in her backpack something I would call *daily-intimate-conversation.* I had what I would have called, at the time, *occasional-debates-about-personal-viewpoints.* Sort of like the people that participate in the show *Naked and Afraid,* they usually agree that water is important, but one might choose a knife as their only tool, while the other chooses a fire-starting kit.

The main feature of this lifelong backpacking trip called "marriage" was that, instead of carrying our own pack, full of the things that we believed we needed for ourselves, we would switch backpacks. From now on, I would carry all of Joanna's relational "needs," and she would carry mine. What a beautiful picture that was in my mind. How romantic! I will be the fulfiller of your needs and you will be the fulfiller of mine. Can a sweeter metaphor of true, lifelong love be created?

Until...

After a while, it becomes extremely difficult trying to be everything that the other person wants you to be, especially since you can't.

So, like a real backpacking trip, you start off so very optimistic, full of energy and excitement... this load is totally doable! This is going to be great fun!

Less than a year into our marriage, I talked to Joanna into moving from Texas to Colorado, mostly so that I would have a better backpacking environment. By the time we had met each other, I had climbed five of the fifty-three fourteeners in Colorado (mountains with an elevation of at least fourteen thousand feet). My hope was that I would conquer them all by the time I was thirty.

The first fourteener I climbed was the most difficult physical activity I had ever participated in. I have run more than thirteen miles, without stopping, numerous times. But this made those runs look easy. It was a four-day, three-night ordeal. You drive to the trailhead and park. That's where the wilderness starts—no more vehicles, electricity, or plumbing, no man-made structures, just hundreds of square miles of pristine wilderness with hiking trails. You load your pack with what you think you will need for the next few days and off you go. Your pack weighs about sixty pounds but you're excited, so it doesn't seem that heavy. The first hour or two is relatively easy... you're hiking alongside the creeks and streams. But then, the trail begins to take an unnatural direction. Instead of following the main water sources, it abruptly turns uphill, toward the summit. When you left your vehicle, you were at about six thousand feet above sea level. Your destination is another eight thousand feet higher. To put it in perspective, that's the equivalent of climbing a ladder that is over a mile and a half high. That's six Empire State buildings or eight Eifel Towers. Pushing yourself uphill with this much weight on your back, you will need at least three times as much oxygen, but there is only about half as much available oxygen as there is at sea level. You won't make the summit today, maybe not even tomorrow, if you're not yet acclimated to the altitude.

You begin to notice, more and more, that you're working extremely hard. You're now gaining only a foot of altitude with every few steps. After ten or fifteen minutes of this, no matter how slow you are taking it, you will have to stop and rest. That's when you take your backpack off. You've got to have some relief of this burden. The shoulder straps are digging in to the sides of your neck, causing a sharp pain. Your hips are screaming "this ain't right." Your entire body is yelling "we need relief!"

So, you take off your pack, sit down on a fallen tree or rock, and set your pack next to yourself, leaning it against whatever you're sitting on. The first thing you do is reach for your water bottle. You catch your breath between gulps, and, after a few minutes, your heart rate slows down to a manageable level. That's when you open your pack. You look to see if there's something you're carrying that you don't need to carry.

I ask myself, "Do I really need this gallon of Gatorade?" I had been fantasizing about what a hit I would be to the group when we finally reached the summit, exhausted, head pounding from altitude sickness, dying of thirst, and I would break out the Gatorade for everyone to feast upon. Not only would they be falling all over themselves to thank me, they would express their admiration of me for carrying an extra 8.35 pounds, for two days, twenty-four thousand steps, for the sole purpose of helping the group regain desperately needed hydration, carbohydrates, and electrolytes. I would be a hero! I would be accepted.

Right there and then, on the very first day, two hours into the four-day hike, I swigged down half of the Gatorade, leaving noticeable traces of my parched and gummed-up mouth around the opening of the bottle and announcing, "does anyone want some Gatorade?" A few desperate individuals took a swig, without a sign of gratitude as they focused on a tree in the distance, so as to avoid thinking about the "salty crusties" left behind by my sticky mouth. It wasn't my plan for this fine vintage of original lemon-lime flavored Gatorade, but at least I didn't half to heave it the rest of the way up the mountain.

A few months into our marriage, something similar happened on our lifelong backpacking trip together: We enjoyed the first few months of the new adventure together, carrying each other's packs. But then, real life set in. We had to start thinking seriously about paying the bills, dividing up domestic duties in a way we both deemed fair and reasonable, and, most importantly, dealing with someone who did backpacking (marriage and life in general) different from ourselves. We had now detoured off the easy path onto the path that mattered most: the path toward what we each believed really mattered for life—the summit.

We had talked about it enough to know that we both wanted the same basic things: a commitment to a life together as long as we both lived, children, a shared faith, and basic values. So, we were both headed toward the same summit. But now we were discovering that we both had very different ideas of how we get to that summit. Sometimes those differences were about one of us thinking the North face was the best, while the other thought the South approach was safer. But more of the day-to-day differences were about the smaller details: whether to hike hard and fast and take several breaks or to go slow and steady and take few breaks and whether to camp near a stream so that water would be more available or to camp away from water sources so that dangerous animals, which hang out close to water, wouldn't be as much of an issue. A loose translation: whether we should spend more of our money enjoying today or saving it for an even better thing in the future. Do we live in a diverse culture where the children will be exposed to differences that will often prove more difficult to navigate but help instill more understanding and compassion, or do we live in a more homogenous culture that more accurately reflects and encourages our way of thinking?

So, after we get a short distance along this steeper and more uncertain terrain, we noticed it was time to stop and rest.

That's when we each took off the pack on our back, which was actually the other person's pack that we were so romantically carrying. After catching our breath, we open that pack up to see if there is something in there that we don't *really* need. And, of course, since we are *not* carrying our own pack, we notice several things in there that we don't believe we really need, though the other one does. I look into Joanna's pack and see *daily-intimate-conversation*. Right away I think to myself, "Really? Daily? Intimate? We don't need that!"

So, as I'm pulling it out of the pack, I'm hoisting it up like a gallon of Gatorade as I exclaim, "This is good, but we don't really need it and I don't think I have the strength to carry it to the summit anyway. Did you know this weighs 8.35 pounds? And that's not including the glass jar!"[1]

At the same moment, Joanna is looking into my pack and notices *frequent-and-exciting-sexual-intimacy*. As she lifts it out of *my* pack, which she has been carrying, she responds with, "You think *that* is an unnecessary item, look at *this*! It is so unrealistic for you to believe that anyone could provide their spouse with frequent and exciting sex, day after day, week after week, month after month and, assuming your body and mind could take on such superhuman endeavors, would be so miraculously married to that one person who would treat them in such a way that they would even want to! We don't need this for our journey. I'm not carrying it anymore!"

But then we give each other a look that says, "This is what you signed up for. You're supposed to fulfill my needs. Put that back in the pack, and, by golly, you better be thankful when you remember that you have the privilege of carrying that for me!"

And so, the resentments begin to settle in. And, as they do, we begin

---

[1] **In the 1980s Gatorade came in a glass jar.**

to believe that the backpack we are carrying is heavier than the one they are carrying, that it has more unnecessary weight than the other. We also begin to resent when the other doesn't seem to appreciate this huge sacrifice we are making, just for their sake.

Up until just a few years ago, I would always carry this little bag of spices in my pack. It had all sorts of things like cumin, garlic, oregano, parsley, sage, rosemary, and thyme. Also, a picture of Simon and Garfunkel. Just kidding. There was no picture of Simon and Garfunkel. That was just to wake you up in case your mind was wandering.[2] My idea was that I was going to help our wilderness meals taste gourmet. Everyone would be so thankful that I brought along these spices, and, again, I would be the hero of the moment. The thing is, those spices have been used maybe once. After hiking uphill for five hours with sixty pounds on your back, you can eat beans straight out of a can, and it will taste like the best meal you've had in weeks. Not to mention, you're way too exhausted to mess with spices. A lot of things we carry around in our relational packs, because we think they will make the relationship better, only weigh us down. Imagine if, all those years, I was demanding someone else carry that bag of spices that nobody ever used. It wouldn't be long before I hear a frustrated, "Carry them yourself if you want them!"

So, we often are weighing ourselves and our partners down with unneeded weight. But that's not so much the problem as who is being expected and required to carry it. Joanna and I had to finally realize that we needed to switch packs and carry our own weight. But first we had to admit to ourselves and each other that we don't have the ability to carry each other's wants, desires, and needs. I can't be everything she needs. She can't be everything I need. It's an unbearable burden.

Now, this doesn't mean that we don't sometimes carry something for the other person. And, sometimes we may have to carry their whole pack

---

[2] In 1966, Paul Simon and Art Garfunkel released their third album *Parsley, Sage, Rosemary And Thyme*. It included a hit song by the same title. If you don't know who Simon and Garfunkel are, you're missing out on some great tunes! Joanna would say otherwise.

while also carrying our own. If I am really struggling through a particularly stressful time with my work, for example, Joanna will step up her game and go the extra mile to take on some of my chores or be extra considerate of my frayed nerves. When her mother died, we went through a season where I had to stretch myself to be more patient and understanding than usual. But what helped us both to take on those extra loads for a temporary time was knowing that the other didn't require it of us, that they saw it as an act of love, not a fulfillment of an obligation. And that attitude makes all the difference in the world when it comes to finding the strength, patience, compassion, and love that it takes to go above and beyond.

Another way of saying all of this is that we each had to make the decision to free each other from being responsible for our happiness. When we free our spouse from being responsible for our relational fulfillment, we actually begin to create an environment that makes them *want* to do more loving things for us. On the other hand, if we expect them to be the main source of our fulfillment, then when they do something loving for us, it is out of obligation because it's required. And our attitude toward them is, "well that's what you're supposed to do. You're my spouse." We don't appreciate the loving act and they don't feel appreciated, which leaves them increasingly weary of trying to please us in the first place. However, when I free my mate from being responsible for my relational fulfillment and then she does something loving toward me, I see it as a gift. I am thankful. And, I show appreciation, making her want to do more loving things for me. Then we begin to see this profound paradox that so many will miss out on for the rest of their lives: The less I require and expect love from others, the more love I get. The more I expect my mate to fulfill me, the less I am fulfilled.

THE PURSUIT
OF CRAPPINESS

THE PURSUIT OF CRAPPINESS

Happiness is a butterfly, which when pursued, is always just beyond your grasp, but which, if you will sit down quietly, may alight upon you. (**Nathaniel Hawthorne**)

There is another very important piece to this and that's the whole idea of happiness. First, let me state clearly that I'm all for happiness. Call it irony or whatever, but when I'm happy, that's when I'm happiest. That said, I believe the pursuit of happiness is not only a colossal waste of time, it actually makes us *less* happy!

If you think about the way most people refer to personal happiness these days, we should consider how the term is most often used and heard:

"Your happiness is the most important thing."

"If you're not happy with your job, you should do something else."

"I just want to be happy."

"I'm not happy about the way things turned out."

"I'm just not happy in this relationship."

There's a common theme in all these statements: being happy is about circumstances. In other words, being happy is about the things that are happening around us: relationships, coworkers, possessions, weather, traffic, and so on… things outside of us. By any of those measures, things outside of us must be to our liking for us to be happy. If I'm happy because I'm enjoying a beautiful, sunny day at the beach with my family, then

I'm *unhappy* if a sudden thunderstorm blows in. If I'm happy because I'm running a few minutes earlier than scheduled, then I'm *unhappy* if I suddenly run into a traffic jam. If I'm happy because I just opened a letter with an unexpected check for five hundred dollars, then I'm *unhappy* when the next envelope I open has an unexpected bill for six hundred dollars. With this mindset, we are only truly happy when more desired things are happening to us than undesired things. Right now, I desire being served steak and lobster while sunning on a yacht in the Caribbean. None of that may ever happen. So, the pursuit of happiness becomes a striving for more and more ways to control our environment so that we can have more desired things happen to us than *undesired* things. Just when we find that person that makes us happy, they do something that makes us unhappy. So, we try to change them to make us happy again, which makes them unhappy because we aren't accepting them. So, *they* try to change *us* so that they will be happy again, which makes us even less happy, and the cycle continues. When we quit trying to change the other person, we become *more* happy. Put more simply, the less we pursue happiness, the happier we are.

2001 was an extraordinary year for me. Two big things happened that directly affected my life, although each of them happened more than a thousand miles away from me. The first was the earthquake that hit El Salvador and killed hundreds of people on January 13. The second was on September 11, when terrorists hijacked several planes, two of which hit the World Trade Center in New York. Because of my counseling and therapy background, I was invited to be part of two separate teams that went into these two situations to offer help. The first was El Salvador.

When we got to the capital city of San Salvador, the locals that we were connected to informed us that there were already many large, international relief efforts focused on the main city. However, many of the more remote, rural areas were being neglected because of their smaller population and distance from the city. A couple of those locals were already invested in helping bring education and services to one of these smaller villages named "El Sunza." When I say "smaller," it was a village of about six thousand people in an area about the size of eight football fields, about 800 people living on each football field, in houses that were made of dried mud bricks. The average house was about ten feet by ten feet with dirt floors. Few people had electricity. There was no running water or plumbing, and the sewer system was a network of shallow ditches running down the middle of the paths between the houses. Water was retrieved by buckets and jugs from the river which was about a ten-minute walk down the hill. When we arrived, the first thing I noticed was the overwhelming odor of the open sewer system. About one out of every ten houses had collapsed from the earthquake, leaving those families with only tarps for shelters. It had been over a week since the main quake, but nightly aftershock tremors left everyone too afraid to rebuild their homes, concerned that they would just crumble again. We figured out that we could build them new homes with quake-resistant materials, for about a thousand dollars apiece, in about three days per house. We had raised enough money to purchase materials for seven houses. We spent the next six days building the first two houses with them, to show them how the simple design and materials worked together.

Despite all these hardships, these families were the most joyful people I had ever been around. I think much of their joy came from that grateful attitude they seemed to continually display. One overwhelming example of this was one of their sons, David. David was about ten years old. On the first day, he was assigned to be my "assistant," helping me carry water up from the river to mix with the cement, holding the level on the poles while I aligned them, and handing me screws as I fastened the siding. David had only one toy: five marbles of different sizes and colors. It was apparent that none of them had come from the same bag but had been acquired here and there, one as a gift, another found in the bushes. As we parted on that last day, David gave to me his only toy, those five marbles. I still have them in a box on my desk, as a reminder of what it looks like to live joyfully out of gratitude.

Later that year, I spent five days in the huge tent that was set up by The Salvation Army, next to Ground Zero. The entire area had been walled off from the public with a chain-link fence that was about twelve feet high and was covered with material to keep people from seeing in. The only way to get in and out was through the tent, which was equipped with a huge cafeteria and resting stations for the people who were working to clear the sight, most of whom were New York City Police and Firefighters.

My job was to be available as a counselor to anyone one who requested it. There were probably thirty round tables in that tent, with chairs all around them. The main purpose for the tables was for people to eat at during their meal breaks. Meals were being served 24/7 as the site was constantly busy, all day and night. They put me at one of the many tables that was in a corner, with a little, folded paper sign that said "Counselor." I tried to explain that this was a bad idea. People aren't likely to sit down at my table, in plain sight of dozens of others, even if they were desperate for counseling. The stigma of even going to a counselor behind a closed door, in a private practice, is enough to keep many people from getting the help they need.

That first day, nobody came to me for counseling, although almost everyone, who came through, noticed me there with my sign in front of me. So, the next day I switched tactics. When I went through the cafeteria line, I brought my tray out to the *middle* table. After I finished eating, I left my tray in front of me so as to appear that I'm still having breakfast. It wasn't long before I had several firefighters sitting around me, asking me questions, mostly about me and the circumstances that occurred for me to have this privilege. But, over time they began to feel comfortable with me and some of them began to open up a bit. The next three days, I did the same thing. As people were taking their meal breaks, more and more of them would plop their tray down on my table and talk about how 9/11 was affecting their lives.

On the last day, a higher-ranking policeman sat down. After we talked awhile, he asked me if I'd seen the site yet. I showed him the badge they had issued me. It had my picture and said "counselor" on it but nothing to indicate that I was allowed to go through the heavily secured checkpoint at the other end of the tent.

"I'm the one in charge of that checkpoint," he told me. "Would you like to see Ground Zero?"

I answered "No" and that I'm not really into seeing things like that.

Are you awake? Just checking.

Are you crazy? Of course, I answered "YES"!

Actually, "YES" in all caps was what I was thinking inside. But I didn't want to seem excited about seeing a place where 2,606 people had just died, some of whom were his friends and coworkers. But I *was* excited. This was a chance to see the site that I knew would come to represent a moment in history that changed the world forever. He was giving me the opportunity to see it before it was cleaned up, sanitized, and turned into a museum and tourist attraction. I wanted to experience the gravity of it, to see firsthand how twisted ideologies can do actual damage and cause mass suffering. Yes, I was excited and somber and humbled and awed and sickened and intrigued and so on.

As we passed from the site of the fallen World Trade Center into the tent, we walked through a chamber that would disinfect your HAZMAT suit and oxygen mask before you remove them. After walking around the site and looking into that giant hole, which had now been cleared down about thirty feet, I had even more questions. As we removed the yellow HAZMAT suits, I asked him, "How has this changed you?" His answer surprised me.

"This may sound weird to you, but I think it's made me a happier person."

He went on, "Even though I lost some friends and every day I see more body parts removed from that hole, I have come to realize that I need to be thankful for what I *didn't* lose. I mean truly thankful. The kind of thankful you are when someone has gone out of their way to do something for you. But I'm learning to be that sort of thankful all the time, because you never know when some of it might be taken away from you, a piece of your community, a friend, your sense of security and safety, and so on. Before all this happened, I wouldn't have taken the time to sit down by a counselor who looks like a lonely fish out of water, much less talk to you. But my new state of gratitude has made me happier and given me a desire to pass my joy on to others."

The policeman and little David, in El Salvador, were stark reminders of what we can experience when we quit pursuing happiness, when we instead choose to be grateful for what we *do* have and live each day as if it could be taken away from us tomorrow, and when we quit focusing on what we wish was different about our mate and, instead, be thankful for what is good about her or him.

If you are going to be happy in your marriage, you must first realize that the source of your unhappiness is not your spouse. Let me say this in another way: If you can't be happy being married to your spouse, then you won't be happy *not* being married to your spouse. If your relationship with your spouse is what is dictating your happiness, or lack thereof, that means that your spouse dictates your well-being. External circumstances are the things that are robbing you of joy. So, if you switch to a different set of external circumstances, those circumstances will also eventually let you down, leaving you unhappy again.

A landmark study looked at over 1,500 couples. Those who reported as being unhappy in their marriage, so they got a divorce, were no happier five years later. The majority were actually less happy.[1] They believed that it was their spouse's behavior that dictated their happiness. In other words, they believed that their happiness was the result of something outside of themselves. So, they took that mindset with them and applied it to their next relationship or marriage.

Now, I know that some people are really messed up and very toxic. They make it difficult for anyone to have a good marriage with them. Unless they start learning how to love, their spouses are going to struggle to maintain a good relationship with them. I have a friend who is married to someone like that. We'll call him Anthony.

Anthony is not a close friend. I only see him a few times a year, but

---

[1] **Does Divorce Make People Happy? Findings from a Study of Unhappy Marriages By Linda J. Waite, Don Browning, William J. Doherty, Maggie Gallagher, Ye Luo, and Scott M. Stanley, 2002**

he is a good friend of one of my good friends who we will call Eric. Most of my interaction with Anthony is during an annual three-day couples retreat that Joanna and I have been attending for almost twenty years. So, each year during those three days, I get to see quite a bit about how Anthony and his wife interact. Now Anthony is a very likeable guy. But his wife seems to me like a person that would be difficult to love. She often berates him and talks harshly to him in public. I should also say that she does the same to others as well. A couple of years ago, I was talking with our mutual friend Eric when, for some reason I don't recall, the subject of Anthony and his wife came up.

"Man," I said to Eric. "I feel sorry for Anthony. It must be very hard to love a wife like his."

To this Eric replied, "What do you mean? Anthony adores his wife! They get along great!"

This statement of Eric's was very convicting to me. It made me wonder how often someone had said something similar about what a wonderful person Joanna must be for putting up with me all these years. Anthony, like Joanna, has learned that he can be happy and joyful regardless of how his spouse behaves. On top of that, he can actually have a great relationship with her. He has learned one of the great secrets to lifelong love. He has freed his spouse from being responsible for his happiness.

Although I liked the movie *Jerry Maguire*, there is a particular scene that most people remember when Tom Cruise tells Renée Zellweger, "You complete me." When I first saw that movie, over two decades ago, I thought that it was one of the most romantic statements I had ever heard. But about five years ago, I went to hear Gary Smalley speak. Gary died a few years ago, but he left a legacy of being one of the top marriage specialists in the world, along with several best-selling books. In that speech he said that one of the most romantic things you can tell your spouse is "I *don't* need you."

You read that correctly. But there was a pause after he said that and then he finished the statement.

"But I *want* you."

Dr. Smalley was emphasizing this point: if we are incomplete *without* our spouse, we will be incomplete *with* our spouse. Two half-healthy people together don't make a whole healthy marriage. Two half-healthy people together make each other sicker. If I have a cold and you have the flu, we shouldn't be hanging around each other.

If I rely on another person to complete me, then I will also buy into the idea that marriage is a fifty-fifty proposition, an equation doomed to disaster. You see, if I'm only trying to give fifty percent, I will almost always fall short of meeting that. I will make mistakes. I will often only be thinking of my own wants and needs. So, on my best days, I'm going to only be doing about thirty percent. Assuming my spouse is a human who is likewise thinking more about her own wants and needs than mine, on a good day we're going to achieve sixty percent together, not even a passing grade. On the other hand, if I'm continually striving for 100%, even if I'm only hitting seventy percent consistently, my spouse only needs to hit twenty percent consistently for our marriage to get an "A." This is the secret that Anthony had learned.

Two of the best-selling marriage books of the last few decades are *His Needs, Her Needs* by Willard Harley and *The Five Love Languages* by Gary Chapman. I personally think they are very helpful books. I continue to refer to them in courses I teach. These two books have had a great impact on our culture. Even people who have never read either of these books or are even familiar with the names of the authors will say things like, "She doesn't meet my needs" or "He doesn't speak my love language." Before these two books came along, those phrases were not common to our culture.

I hope that this book helps a lot of people. But I hope it does *not* result in people saying things like, "If you accept me, you accept my alcohol abuse" or "Why can't you accept the fact that I have sex with other partners?" Accepting a person does not mean accepting their behavior. We *should* be getting better and better at speaking the *love language* of our spouse and meeting more and more of their relational *needs*. But to expect that your spouse is going to be able to meet all your needs or be fluent in your love language is to set yourself up with expectations that can never be met. You want to be happier? Repeat these three mantras every day:

No one can meet all my needs.
No one can speak my love language fluently.
No one is going to fully accept me.

Christmas of 2018 looked like it would be Glen McCarthy's last. Homeless, Glen was living in a run-down hotel in Denver, Colorado. Glen was dying of terminal cancer and had very little money left to his name. So, he walked to Walmart with what little he had left. Remembering that there was a bin set up, at Walmart, for people to buy toys and donate them to less fortunate children for Christmas, Glen bought a Barbie and some Hot Wheels. Then he noticed a bicycle that had two price tags on it. One price tag was for $59, and the other, which looked like it didn't belong on the bike, was for $44. He didn't have enough money left over for the $59 price, but he had enough for the $44 price. Glen thought about how happy that bike would have made him when he was a child. He asked to talk to a manager.

He convinced the manager to give it to him for the $44 price since he intended to donate it. Glen said that it took losing everything he had to realize that he is happier now—when he has to think of every dollar— than when he had "big money." Why do so many of us learn this lesson so late in life and some of us never learn it? I'm hoping to learn it sooner than later!

Why You Like Your Spouse Or, Why You Don't Like Your Spouse

Why You Like Your Spouse Or, Why You *Don't* Like Your Spouse

How you think about your spouse has more to do with what *you* do than what *he* or *she* does. Also, how you feel about your spouse has more to do with what *you* do than what she or he does. Let me put this in another way: your attitudes and feelings, about your spouse, are mostly affected by your own actions. Of all the concepts I teach, this one seems to be the most difficult for people to grasp. It seems so counterintuitive to so many. Yet it is vitally important that you begin to adopt this way of being if you want to have any hope of lifelong love.

If you are having trouble considering this idea, it may be because you know of things that your significant other does or fails to do, which makes it harder for you to like them or have pleasant thoughts and feelings about them. While it is true that others' actions *influence* our thoughts and feelings toward them, that influence is not as strong as our *own* attitudes and actions. Let's look at a real-life example: tarantulas.

Tarantulas are big, hairy spiders with fangs and are venomous. That much most of us know. Imagine a group of six people, randomly chosen from the population, sitting around a table when, suddenly, someone walks in and throws a live tarantula in the middle of that table. About once a month, I conduct a three-day intensive workshop for marriages. When I am introducing the concept of this chapter, I take a poll. I ask each person in the room what their reaction would be to this scenario of a live tarantula being thrown in front of them onto this table. There are basically three different answers:

1. Jump up and run away (usually with some sort of screaming involved)
2. Lean or scoot back a bit
3. Lean in and attempt to touch it or even let it walk on their arm

Of those three basic answers, numbers 1 and 2 are what about eighty-five percent report as how they would react. That leaves about fifteen percent who report reaction number 3: lean in and attempt to touch it or even let the tarantula walk on their arm. So, why do we have three very different reactions to the same scenario? Does the tarantula think to itself "Today I'm going to intentionally scare forty-five percent of the humans I encounter out of the room. To another forty percent, I'm going to do just enough to make them respect me with a little space. And, for fifteen percent of the humans I meet today, I will do my best to make friends with"? Of course not! It's not the tarantula that decides how we think and feel about it, it's our own beliefs and attitudes that most affect how we think and feel toward the tarantula.

Where do these attitudes and beliefs come from? Why do they vary so sharply between group one and group three? It's because of the difference in experiences between those two groups. In other words, it's what they have done in their lives. If your only experience with tarantulas has been to watch movies like *Arachnophobia* and hang around people who *have* arachnophobia, you are likely to be in group one, and your emotional and physical reaction (how you think and feel about the tarantula) would be to run out of the room in terror. Myself, on the other hand, would be part of group three. I would place one hand, palm down, on the table, in front of the tarantula. And, I would use the other hand to gently coax it up on to my hand.

Now, let me be clear. There was a time when I would have been in group 1 or 2. However, when I was teenager, my school class took a field trip to the zoo. That day we did the usual tour of all the animals that were on display. But, toward the end of the visit, the guide brought us all into a laboratory where he brought out different animals that were safe enough to handle. One of them was a boa constrictor that was about three feet long. As he held it, he gave a short lecture on boas and how they were not venomous and the best ways to handle them. He then asked if anyone would volunteer to handle it themselves. My hand was the first to go up. You see, I was always one of the smallest boys at school. This has had a lot to do with one of my insecurities which some would refer to as a "Napoleon complex." I was always trying to prove that I was at least as tough and courageous as anyone else. My wife says I still do this. She's probably correct. So, I handled the boa in front of all my classmates as I imagined that all the girls were so impressed with me that they were dreaming of me asking them to dance at the next school-sponsored banquet.

After a few minutes, he took the boa back from me, put it back in its box, and brought out a live tarantula. Again, as he let the tarantula walk from one of his arms to the other, he explained that while tarantulas *are* venomous, the venom is no more potent than the average bee sting. Furthermore, they rarely bite people and no one on record has ever been known to die of a tarantula bite. On top of that, a tarantula's first line of defense is to run away. If they can't get away, they will next drop some of the hairs from their belly and try to kick them at you. They don't want to bite you. They are afraid of you. They want you to leave them alone. But, once they feel safe that you are not going to stomp them to death, they will happily coexist with you.

After explaining all of this, again, he asked if anyone wanted to let the tarantula walk on their arm. Although my hand went up first again, I was much more nervous this time. As he approached me, my heart rate went way up, and adrenaline began flooding my neurons. But, after a few moments with the spider calmly sitting on my arm, I began to calm down and my heart rate returned to normal. As I handed the tarantula back to the zookeeper and glanced around the room, it seemed as if my school-yard cred had just shot up 100% percent.

I had seen tarantulas on the road in front of our house from time to time. So that day, when I got home, I went out into the field and hunted until I found two live tarantulas. I brought them home and put them into an old empty aquarium, a remnant of a tropical fish experiment, which my little brother and I had undertaken, gone wrong. Every day I would take them out and practice handling them with more and more ease. I was really going to impress the ladies now, so I thought.

Just like our reactions to tarantulas are mostly influenced by our own actions rather than the tarantula's actions, so too are our thoughts and feelings toward our mate.

But you may be thinking to yourself, "That's animals. But we're talking about relationships—relationships between humans!"

So, let me illustrate this with a human-to-human example. This example, by the way, is just one of many real-life examples I could give you. It begins with a guy I'll call *Henry*, to protect his identity. Henry came to me seeking help for depression. His wife had been deceased for two years. He explained to me that early on he thought he was just going through normal grieving, but now, two years later, he still breaks down crying several times a day, sometimes sobbing so much that he has to pull his car over because he can't see clearly through the tears. Furthermore, he was having trouble just having enough will just to get out of bed each morning. "I still miss her so much," he told me.

That first session, he also brought along two spiral notebooks. "I want you to see these, so you get an idea of how much I loved her," he said. I thumbed through the second one enough to notice that it was filled with daily entries that he had written about her. It was like a daily journal, with the date at the beginning of each entry, except the entries were only about his wife, nothing else and nobody else. I also noticed that the dates on each entry began about three years prior to that session and ended about two years prior, the final year of his wife's life. Then it came to an abrupt stop. She died and he quit journaling about her.

"Why did you decide to keep this journal?" I asked.

He then explained that his wife had died of a severe form of cancer. By the time she was diagnosed, the cancer had spread and become inoperable. She would not likely live more than a year. When Henry heard this from the doctor, he was secretly glad. He didn't like his wife. They had been married for over forty years, and, as those years passed, he had become increasingly resentful toward her. He had reached a point where his thoughts and feelings toward her were so negative he was now looking forward to spending the rest of his life without her.

After of a few days of looking forward to his wife's death, he began to feel guilty, so much so that he confided in a trusted and respected friend. The friend recommend that he go out that very day and buy a spiral notebook, open it up to the first page, write the date at the top, and then write at least one thing about her for which he is grateful. "Do this every day," he told Henry. So, Henry did.

At this point in our session, I picked up the first spiral notebook and opened it to the first page. That first day's entry had the date and then two words: "good cook."

That was it. That was all he could come up with for the first day. But as I thumbed through the first notebook and into the second, I noticed that the entries were getting longer and longer. Toward the end of that last year of her life, in journal number two, many of the entries were several pages long and looked as if they were penned by a lovestruck poet. I looked up at him as I finished reading one of the last entries. My eyes were getting teary.

"Wow, it looks like going through cancer really changed her," I said.

"No," he responded. "She was always a wonderful lady. It's just that, over the years I began to focus, more and more, on the things I didn't like about her. Doing this journal turned my focus back to the things that are good about her. That shift in focus, reframing how I chose to see her, changed *me*!"

What *we* do has much more to do with how we think and feel about our mate than what our mate does.

Most of the things that irritate us about our mate were there before we met them. They may even be things that actually attracted us to them in the first place. As I noted earlier, I come out on the introvert side of most personality assessments. My wife, on the other hand, is off-the-charts extroverted. She is one of the most warm, friendly, and talkative people you will meet. Not only did I know this about her when I first met her, it was one of the main things that attracted me to her. So, we started dating, fell in limerence, and got married. Like most married couples, we then moved in together. We got a little apartment, and, right away, we began to notice things about each other that we wanted to change. She liked lamp-lit rooms instead of ceiling lights. I preferred the ceiling lights because they were easy to turn on and off by the switch on the wall. She felt ignored and unloved when I refused to use the lamps. I wanted to display my rock collection in the living room. She saw absolutely no decorative value in a bright yellow chunk of pure sulfur. I felt dismissed and unloved when she refused to let me put my rock collection on the bookshelf. As these sorts of things occurred, the limerence began to fade. As the limerence began to fade, we both tried bringing it back by changing each other. As we tried to change each other (the opposite of acceptance), we felt even less loved and began to resent each other. As I began to resent Joanna, I began seeing everything about her in a negative light, including her gift of gab. As I told myself more and more, "she talks too much," I noticed it even more and began resenting the very thing that I fell in love with in the first place.

Every great personality feature has its dark side. My personality is to seek peace and harmony with others. One of the dark sides of a personality like that is that I am also prone to avoid conflict. But someone who avoids conflict will have even more conflict in the long run because they will often sweep difficult issues under the rug, hoping they just go away.

Instead, they lie under the rug, rotting and molding until they become even bigger issues than they were in the first place. But, eventually, Joanna and I decided we had to make every effort to focus on the "light" side of each other's personalities. I had to make it a point, every day, to be thankful for her talkative nature. She had to do the same about my desire for peace and harmony. When we focus on the dark side of our mate's personality features, we plant a seed of bitterness that will grow into an overwhelming briar patch, as long as we keep feeding it.

Back when I was watering and fertilizing my bitterness toward Joanna's talking, I was having lunch one day with a friend who was older and wiser and cared about my marriage. During that lunch he asked me how my marriage was going. At this point we had been married about three years. I told him that I was really frustrated with Joanna because it seemed like she talks constantly.

He replied, "She's been talkative ever since I've known her. Wasn't she talkative when you met her?"

"Yeah, I guess she was," I said.

"So, it's probably something that attracted you to her in the first place," he said.

"I have to admit you're right, but it seems like it's increased since I met her," I said.

To which he replied, "I highly doubt that. It's more likely that you have chosen to focus on that as a *negative* about her. When we get focused on something negative, it becomes even more negative in our minds. Jon, since you are a person of prayer, I want you to make sure you pray, at least once a day, thanking God that Joanna loves to talk."

To which I replied, "That would be dishonest. I couldn't pray that and really mean it."

"Oh yes you can," he said. "You just have to put a different frame around the way you look at her talkative nature. When you were dating Joanna, you framed her as outgoing, warm, friendly, gregarious, and able to talk to anyone and make them feel like they mattered. Over time, you tore that frame up and began to build a frame of *annoying, loud, chatterbox*. Just start thanking God about the light side of that personality trait. Oh, by the way, you have a lot of friends because Joanna is so out-going. People assume you must be a great guy because you're married to such a great gal. So, you could also thank God that you have more friends because of her talkative nature."

Within a couple of months of daily thanksgiving for Joanna's talking, I began to see that aspect again like I did in the beginning. He was right. How I think and feel toward my mate has more to do with what *I* do than what *she* does!

This chapter is so crucial to having lifelong love that I am going to close with one more perspective.

What do you think and how do you feel about the President of the USA? It doesn't matter which one. Just pick one of the last three. How do you think and feel about him? Well, roughly half the population thinks and feels the opposite. Why? Most of us have never met him, much less ever been in the same room with him. It is likely that you have never been in any direct contact with him. Yet, you have strong thoughts and feelings about him, and roughly half Americans have the opposite thoughts and feelings. It's not what the President has done to you that creates most of those attitudes. It's what you've done. If you have hung around people who don't like the President, you're going to like the President less. If you have chosen to get your news from a source that tends to favor the President's party, you're going to like him more. When he signs a bill, millions of people love him for it, and millions loathe him for it. Does his action *influence* those sentiments? Of course! But not near as much as what all those people have been doing, themselves and individually, up to that point.

Blowing Off Steam Or Building Up Gas?

Blowing Off Steam Or
Building Up Gas?

There's a guy named Russell that I've known since seventh grade. We went to junior high and church together. In high school we started to become close friends. Then we went to the same college together and even roomed together in a little dump of an apartment. When things began to get more serious with Joanna, Russell asked me if I was going to marry her. I told him that I probably will, if she'll have me. Then I added that Joanna's sister, Gina, was only six months older than him, even though she was a year ahead of us in school, and that he should marry her so we could keep hanging out together for the rest of our lives. So, Russell married Gina about a year after Joanna and I married, just so we could hang out for the rest of our lives. Just kidding. Sort of.

I know… creepy.

As I mentioned before, Joanna and I moved to Colorado about a year after we married. So, Russell and Gina moved to Colorado a few months after us. For five years, Russell and Gina lived in the same apartment complex as Joanna and me. A couple of years, after we moved to Colorado, I started working for the same company Russell worked for. We carpooled to and from work together for the next five years. This was around the time when our marriage had hit its low point and we had grown very frustrated with each other.

Several mornings a week, during our twenty-minute commute to work, Russell would have to hear me complain about Joanna the entire way. This went on for probably a year. One day, while I was in the middle of one of my rants, Russell interrupted.

Russell: "Jon, I don't want to hear it anymore."

Jon: "Okay, enough for today."

Russell: "No. Not for today… for good. I don't want you talking bad about Joanna anymore."

Jon: "I'm just blowing off steam."

Russell: "I don't think you are."

Jon: "I love her, and I'm committed to her. You're the only one I do this with because you know that, and you're my best friend. Best friends are supposed to help their best friends vent!"

Russell: "Well, I don't think it's helping you or your marriage, so I'm not going to listen to it anymore."

I was hurt. I was angry. I thought I was losing a friend or at least being abandoned by a friend. It took me a few days to realize what he was saying:

You don't blow off steam by talking bad about someone. You build gas!

Think about it. When you have been verbally running someone into the ground, do you like them more when you're finished? Of course not. You like them less. So, each time you do it, you're liking them less and less. When you like someone less and less, you're going to treat them worse and worse. And, they are likely to treat you worse and worse as a result. One of the most damaging things you can do for your marriage is to talk negatively about your spouse to others.

Another thing I learned, from that car ride with Russell, is that a good friend cares about your marriage. In other words, a good friend cares about your spouse. Your marriage is your most important human relationship. So, if someone doesn't make your marriage better, they will make it worse. It is impossible for anyone that you associate with to have no influence on your marriage. Their influence is either going to support your marriage or erode it. If they don't support it, they're not a good friend. They don't care about you if they don't care about your most important relationship. Period.

That said, I can go to Russell, to this day, if I'm having a problem with Joanna. He will listen, as long as he can tell that I'm truly asking for help, that I'm coming to him for advice on what *I* can do differently. But, if I'm attempting to make Joanna look bad, especially for the sake of having someone to commiserate with me, then he will gently interrupt and remind me that he doesn't play that game. That's a good friend! And, that's very different from "venting."

Some people have friends or even family members that need the *Russell treatment*. They need to sit down and tell them, "Look. My marriage is the most important human relationship I have. You are either going to be a part of supporting that or you're going to have to *not* be involved in my life. I love you, but I have to love my spouse more." You may have to say that to a friend you've had since before you met your spouse. You may have to say it to a relative. You may even have to say it to one of your parents. If they truly love you, they will come around, eventually. If they don't start supporting your marriage, it may be a sign that they don't really love you but, instead, want to control you.

Now, I know there are exceptions to this. If my child was being sexually or physically abused by his or her spouse, I would attempt to influence my child to get away from him or her. However, just because I don't happen to approve of who my child marries does not give me the right, as a parent, to sabotage that decision, once it's made.

It was years before I realized that both mine and Joanna's parents had been teaching us this lesson from early on. The first year of our marriage, we were still full-time college students. Apart from our classes and homework, we worked just enough to pay the rent and eat very basic food. So, at least once a week, we would go eat at my parent's house, and at least once a week, we would eat at her parent's house so we could get a free meal and eat some of mom's good cooking.

After a few months of living together and trying to change what we thought was wrong about each other, we began to realize that our efforts to change each other weren't working. So, we each thought we needed to call in some reinforcements. When we were sitting around *my* parents' table, I would bring up something that I knew my parents would share my point of view.

Jon: "Joanna thinks eating our chickens is gross because they came from our backyard instead of the grocery store. Would you two set her straight on this matter?"

Jon's Mom: "Well, lots of people don't like the idea of eating something that they saw walking around the day before."

Jon's Dad: "You have to remember, Joanna and her parents grew up in the city. We all grew up on farms and we're just used to it."

What? I knew my parents agreed with my point of view. Our chickens were much cleaner and healthier than the ones from the store that had grown up in a little cramped cage, sitting in their own feces and being pooped on by the chickens above them! (Sorry if I just made you not like chicken anymore but that's how it works with most mass-produced chicken.) But why were they taking *her* side?

Then, a few days later, we would be sitting around the dinner table at Joanna's house. That's when the same dynamic would be flipped in my favor:

Joanna: "Jon doesn't put the toilet seat down when he's finished. His mom didn't teach him right and he won't listen to me."

Joanna's Mom: "Well, Joanna, Jon grew up sharing a bathroom with the males in his family. You grew up sharing a bathroom with the females in your family."

Joanna's Dad: "Joanna, you didn't have any brothers. It took me several years of sharing a bathroom with your mom and all your sisters before I realized that the middle-of-the-night pee is different for boys than it is for girls. Sure, both sexes are half asleep when they get up, but guys don't fall in if the seat is left up."

Joanna: "Why are you taking his side? You know I'm right! Plus, Jon never had to clean his own toilet growing up. People who don't clean toilets don't seem to consider the people who do!"

Joanna's Mom: "I'm sure Jon could say the same about how you don't make sure the oil in your car is changed every three thousand miles."

Now, if you found yourself picking sides on these two issues, you've missed the point entirely. These two illustrations are not about who has the more valid point. They are about a much more important issue: the relationship between Joanna and me. It took me decades to appreciate what I should have been hearing our parents saying back in our first year of marriage: *As your parents, if we are going to be on your side, we are going to be on both of your sides. Don't try to use us against your spouse. If we care about you, we care about your most important human relationship—your marriage.*

Our oldest daughter has been married for over six years now. When she first got engaged, Joanna and I got with her future parents-in-law and threw them an engagement party. One of the things that all of us parents agreed on was that we needed to bless them by letting them know that, from now on, we were going to work together to support their marriage. So, at the party, the four of us stood united in telling our two children that we are now on both of their sides, not on the side of our child, when he or she differs from their spouse. As parents, we are either going to be a part of making our child's life better or worse. There is no in between. If we are not part of strengthening their marriage, we will be a part of making their marriage worse. In fact, as parents, we are probably the people with the *most* influence on their marriage. Rarely is it loving of us to come in between our child and their spouse.

REAL SCIENCE VS. CULTURAL MINDSETS

REAL SCIENCE VS.
CULTURAL MINDSETS

A while back I was checking out a rental car at the Nashville airport. I was on business, so I was paying with my business credit card. The young lady at the counter looked at the credit card and asked me what kind of business this was, so I explained to her that I work with marriages.

Her eyes grew wide. She didn't utter a word but fairly shouted with her look: *Ah hah! At last, someone credible who can confirm that I'm right in my debate with my relative/friend/coworker/significant other.*

Sure enough, she said, "So, let me ask you a question. What do you think about people living together before marriage?"

From that point, I could have written the script. I have an elevator speech for many such topics and wasn't three words in when she interrupted: "Tina! Come listen to this guy. He's a marriage expert. I just asked him what he thought about living together."

Tina, her coworker, sidled down the counter and stood with her arms crossed while a familiar-looking wave of emotions—curiosity? skepticism? hope?—flashed across her face.

Me: "Let me guess. You're both living with someone, but you're not married."

They nodded in unison.

"And your parents are telling you it's wrong."

"Yep."

Me: "Okay, without getting into the moral question, there's a lot of data on the topic. And the scales just don't tip in your favor."

The first young lady spoke: "But that doesn't make sense. You wouldn't buy a car without taking it for a test-drive. Why would you make a life-long commitment to marriage without really knowing what it's like living together?"

I didn't have the time, nor did I think I would have changed their made-up minds in the moment, so I simply replied, "You should Google the research on the subject. You will be very surprised!"

Here is just a sampling of what they would find if they were to do that research:

Cohabitation is usually a short-term arrangement, typically resulting in either marriage or a break-up after about a year (median duration of 1.3 years) (Smith, 2006; Thomson and Colella, 1992; Bumpass and Sweet, 1989).

Marriages formed after cohabitation are rated as less stable and result in more divorces than marriages not preceded by living together (Smith, 2006; Axinn and Thornton, 1992; Brown and Booth, 1996).

Infidelity during marriage is more common among people who lived together prior to marriage than those who did not (Smith, 2006; Forste and Tanfer, 1996).

Cohabiting men are four times as likely as husbands to report infidelity in the past year (Laumann, Gagnon, Michael, and Michaels, 1994; McManus and McManus, 2008).

Cohabiting women are eight times more likely than wives to cheat on their partners (Laumann, Gagnon, Michael, and Michaels, 1994; McManus and McManus, 2008).

People who lived together before marriage have a higher rate of divorce than those who did not live together (Kamp Dush, Cohan, and Amato, 2003).

People who lived together before marriage have more negative communication in their marriages than those who did not live together (Cohan and Kleinbaum, 2002; DeMaris and Leslie, 1984).

People who lived together before marriage have lower levels of marital satisfaction than those who did not live together (DeMaris and Leslie, 1984).

Physical aggression is more common among married individuals who lived together before marriage than those who did not (Stets and Straus, 1989).

60% of those who had cohabited before marriage were more verbally aggressive, less supportive of one another, and more hostile than the 40 % of spouses who had not lived together (Cohan and Kleinbaum, 2002).

In my experience, this example is indicative of the vast majority of our culture. It's not that people don't want to do relationships in a healthy way. People just assume that the cultural norm is intellectually and scientifically superior to all the ways of the past. Instead of keeping what is good from past ways and culling out what is not, we have thrown the baby out with the bath water. We believe that the new mindset and practices are the result of moving toward greater enlightenment.

At the same time, I am not an advocate for "going back to the old ways." Many of the old ways were wrong. For example, it is good that we get away from practicing the sexism of our forefathers. However, much of our "moving forward" is not based on truth, as many would like to believe. A great deal of the way our culture goes about coupling is, at best, making assumptions that are vaguely correlated with empirical evidence and, more often, harmful concepts that have gained credibility simply because so many people are doing them. On the other hand, most of the voices that attempt to counter these harmful practices end up sounding more like irrational fear or clinging to tradition for the sake of tradition. The result is an increasing polarity of two opposing camps that are both losing out because of the blindness that is so often the result of efforts to discredit the other side, instead of trying to learn.

I hope you're reading this book because you truly want to learn how to have better relationships and, even, lifelong love with someone. If so, you will need to assume that most of what you think you know just isn't true. Just because most people are doing it doesn't make it good or right or even more enlightened.

When my children were coming into late elementary or early junior high, I had a conversation with all of them, probably at least three or four times each, that went something like this:

Child Age Eleven: "Dad, can I get a cell phone?"

Dad: "Sure! One day."

Child Age Eleven: "What is that supposed to mean? When I'm grown up?"

Dad: "I don't know. It could probably happen much sooner than that. For example, if you were to buy your own cell phone and make the monthly payments, I think it could happen within the next year!"

Child Age Eleven: "But most of my friends have cell phones that their parents bought for them."

Dad: "Well, your mother and I see things differently than most of your friends' parents."

Child Age Eleven: "But Dad, that's not normal!"

Dad: "I know, but normal sucks!"

If you are striving to be normal, let's take a look at some examples of what you're striving for:

70.2% of North Americans are obese or overweight (National Institute of Diabetes and Digestive and Kidney Diseases, 2018).

Underage Drinking 78% (Journal of the American Medical Association, 2012)

Teen use of Illegal Drugs 42.5% (Journal of the American Medical Association, 2012)

47% of American households have no savings (Business Insider, 2015).

44% of Americans don't have first aid in their home (Wakefield Research, 2018).

The average American-born citizen knows less American History and Civics than Immigrants (Newsweek, 2011).

Being normal should *not* be something to strive for. We must do better than that!

For over forty years, the scientific data has continually and overwhelmingly shown that living together before you decide to marry is a bad idea. Yet, two-thirds of all marriages start with a trial-run marriage called cohabitation.[1] Why do we ignore the facts? Typically, we ignore them when they seem counterintuitive. It makes sense to take a car for a

---

[1] **National Center for Family and Marriage Research, 2011**

test-drive before you buy it. Wouldn't taking a relationship out for a test-drive make sense? Especially in these times when half of all marriages end in divorce!

Except they don't. The divorce rate in North America has never been as high as fifty percent… ever.

In fact, our best estimate is that today, the divorce rate is only about twenty-five percent. That's an overall average. However, there are several demographic factors that put many people below a fifteen percent divorce rate, such as a college degree and attitudes about commitment. So, for most people who marry, the odds are in our favor that the marriage will last as long as the two of us are still alive. One big reason this matters is the influence of fear.

THE FEAR THAT WRECKS RELATIONSHIPS AND MARRIAGE

The Fear that Wrecks Relationships And Marriage

Suppose I could predict, with 100% certainty, whether your spouse would end up leaving you or would stand by you for the rest of their life. Would you want to know? Would it make a difference in that relationship?

Let's look at it in another way: If you were afraid your spouse was eventually going to abandon you, would you treat them differently than if you knew they were always going to accept you as a person and as their spouse? Of course! So would anyone else!

Even if you would like to think that you would consistently act loving toward your spouse, the reality is that our perception has a tremendous amount of influence over our actions, whether we want it to or not. So far, I don't think I will get much intelligent resistance with that line of thinking. But let's keep chasing this rabbit a little further down the trail.

None of us are 100% sure that our spouse will never leave us. Some of us are more sure than others, but none of us can fully rest in the idea that we are, and will always be, totally accepted by our spouse. So, it is safe to say that we all have some degree of the fear of abandonment.

Now think about how these fears play out in day-to-day interaction.

If one of my biggest motivations for choosing a spouse was to be closer to that person than anyone else, to experience true intimacy, emotional and relational and sexual, then I am going to have to make myself vulnerable. However, the more I fear abandonment, the less vulnerable I am going to be. In turn, the less vulnerable I am, the more my spouse will feel abandoned by me.

For example, let's say my spouse wants to engage in more deep conversations with me, but I tend to avoid deep conversations because I might say something that could lead to being rejected. My conversation avoidance leads my spouse to feeling unloved and, in turn, rejected, increasing the likelihood of eventually rejecting me as a spouse. Fear then becomes a self-fulfilling prophecy. **The more we fear rejection, the more we do things that lead to being rejected.**

For several decades now, it has been widely reported that the divorce rate in North America is about fifty percent. This "statistic" has a huge impact on the collective psyche of our culture. If you told me that a huge part of my future was going to be decided by a coin toss, I'm sorry, but I'm not going to totally invest in something that has just as much chance for failure as it does for success. I'm going to keep some things to the side so that I don't lose everything if it lands on "tails." Sign a prenuptial agreement that lets me keep my house? Nah, that would be too obvious! Instead I will spread it out over a bunch of things that don't seem so obvious: I'll invest some of my time, money, energy, emotions, and so on into some safety-net things, activities, and relationships. In other words, I'm not going to *fully* commit to this marriage.

The problem is, if we don't fully commit to the marriage, we simply won't have a good marriage. This is one of the great dilemmas in how our society does relationships. But it doesn't have to be!

So now I must confess, for I have been a contributor to the great American marriage fear factor by quoting many of these dismal "statistics." I haven't been very successful at substantiating them so instead have held the "company line" that about one-half of all marriages end in divorce.

But what if my chances are much better than fifty-fifty? What if there are factors which, if applied, would greatly reduce those chances? Here are some recent findings by researcher and author Shaunti Feldhahn and her team:

The vast majority of marriages are happy.

72 percent of those married are still married to their first spouse.

Of those who report being very unhappy in their marriage, 80 percent report being happily married, just five years later, with that same spouse.

The rate of divorce among those who are active in their faith is significantly lower than the overall average... most likely lower than 10 percent!

According to Shaunti Feldhahn, the divorce rate in the USA has never reached fifty percent. That "statistic" is the result of a projection that was made in the mid-seventies. Since no-fault divorces had recently been adopted by most of the country, divorce rates were rapidly rising. The projection was what they expected, to be in the near future, should the number of divorces continue to rise at the rate they were rising at the time. But the rates leveled off before they ever got that high.[1]

---

[1] By the early 1980s, no-fault divorce was adopted by almost every state in the USA. What this meant for many is that you no longer had to prove that your spouse was sexually unfaithful or physically abusive in order to be granted a divorce. In many ways, this was a great victory for those who found it difficult to prove that they were in an abusive situation, especially women. The State of New York was the last state to adopt no-fault divorce in 1985. One of its main reasons for being a holdout is that it would allow a person to opt out of marriage without incurring the consequences of doing so. A prime example being a husband, with children and a sizeable means of income, could leave his wife bearing the responsibility of raising the children, without his financial support. While there are many pros and cons to the advent of the no-fault divorce, most research has indicated that it has reduced the ability of men to keep their wives in a marriage in which he inflicts physical abuse upon her.

As Feldhahn points out in her recent book, *The Good News About Marriage*, the common denominator behind thriving marriages is **hope**.

When a spouse operates out of fear within the marriage, they tend to do a lot of things that keep the relationship on what I call "relational probation." A marriage on relational probation will never see its potential. Some examples are:

Threatening the relationship with separation or divorce

Withholding affection/love/sex/conversation/approval, in attempt to get the spouse to change (or practically any other reason)

Reinvesting (time, energy, emotions, money) into things other than the marriage

Developing friendships and social structures as a refuge from the marriage

One of the reasons marriages that begin with cohabitation have a higher divorce rate is that many of those marriages started off in fear, although neither one likely recognized the fear. You see, if two people are unsure about committing to marriage, so they move in together to give the relationship a "trial run," they are essentially telling each other, "We'll see how you behave first." The relationship is based on performance instead of acceptance. In other words, they are putting each other on probation from the start. And remember, a relationship on probation will never meet its potential. It will only get worse.

On the other hand, when one operates out of hope, we see more of the following:

Showing more acceptance and less attempts to change the other

Giving love, especially when it isn't deserved

Investing the bulk of their resources into the relationship (like they did when they were dating)

Developing friendships and social structures that have an interest in the marriage

Here's the rub: If you believe that your spouse is acting primarily out of fear, for Peter, Paul, and Mary's sake, don't try to change them! Attempts to do so will only produce more fear that you don't accept them. Instead, love out of hope, and do more and more of the things that made them want to marry you in the first place.

DOES COMMITMENT
REALLY MATTER?

Does Commitment
Really Matter?

When I married Joanna, I knew that I would have to be committed to her, everyone told me so. We all hear that commitment is important in a marriage, don't we? So, it must be, right? We know that commitment is important in marriage because everyone says it is. But do we know what that means?

Going back in time in my head, I'm pretty sure I heard my parents talk to me about commitment in marriage. Since my parents have a loving marriage, and were loving to me, I'm assuming they gave me some sound advice about being a committed husband, although I don't recall any conversations, with either of them, about the topic. Maybe I picked some of my ideas about husbandly commitment from some other married adults as well. I'm sure I did. I just don't recall from whom.

What I *do* remember is that I had two basic ideas of what it meant to be a committed spouse. Those two ideas were:

1. I'm committed to staying married to you.
2. I'm committed to not having sex with anyone but you.

That's pretty much it. That sums up what I thought it meant to be committed to my marriage. As long as I did those two things, I was a committed husband. So, I became very committed to not crossing those two lines so that I could see myself as a committed husband and, hopefully, everyone else would see me that way as well. And then nobody, especially Joanna, could say that I lacked commitment. I was committed to commitment!

Ten years later I'm sitting with one of my first client couples in one of the therapy rooms at the marriage and family therapy clinic at my university. This couple was in their early sixties, married for about forty years, and struggling in their relationship. The wife says to me:

"I just don't think he's committed to me."

Husband: "How can you say that? I have never cheated on you in our forty years, and I have never threatened to divorce you and never will."

Wife: "Is that your definition of commitment... that you won't divorce me and you won't have sex with anyone else?"

Husband: "If that's not commitment to marriage, I don't know what is."

Wife: "I didn't marry you to keep you from divorcing me and having sex with other people. Also, I don't care about your commitment to marriage. I care about your commitment to me!"

Her words, to her husband, struck a huge chord with me. In two sentences she had summed up a giant problem I had in my own marriage. At that moment I realized why my efforts to make Joanna see me as "committed" were failing:

1. I was committed to my principles, not to my spouse.
2. Commitment is more about what we *do*, not what we *don't* do.

Imagine if you were having your annual performance review at work and your boss asked you if you are committed to your job. What would she think if your answer was "I'm committed to not quitting my job, and I'm committed to only taking a paycheck from this company"? There'd better be *way* more to that answer if you plan on keeping that job!

Or, what if your answer was, "Well, I'm somewhat committed"?

Again, that answer is going to put you on the short list for the next round of layoffs. But, my commitment to *not divorcing you* and *not having sex with anyone else* was only *somewhat* of a commitment. Being *somewhat* committed isn't really being committed at all. If you are committed to something, you are *fully* committed to it. So many of the struggling and failing marriages, which I have worked with, have a spouse that is very committed to one or two principles, but not very committed to their spouse. On top of that, they are missing commitment in one or two crucial categories, not realizing that those categories of commitment are crucial to a thriving marriage. Here are the categories that we most often see most missing in a struggling marriage:

Commitment to being there
Commitment to investing in the relationship
Commitment to growth
Commitment to supportive social structures
Commitment to having no alternatives

So, let's look at these, one at a time.

Commitment to Being There

When people decide to marry someone and that someone decides to marry them in turn, there are certain expectations that are normally included in that commitment. When you say, "I do," you believe that the other person is going to be your main "go to" when you want affection, comfort, understanding, or just a shoulder to cry on. The other expects it as well. That's pretty much a given. So, when your spouse wants affection or just to talk about what they're going through in life, you should be their first choice, in most circumstances, as the person who will be there for them. Like the man whose wife said she didn't think he was committed to her, he spent almost all his free time at home with her, but he wasn't committed to being there for *her*. When she wanted someone to talk to about her day, he wasn't willing to turn off the TV for her or set down what he was involved in. He was committed to being there for himself. That's not marital commitment, and although some couples like that may never actually divorce, they don't have much of a marriage. They're just sharing a roof, domestic responsibilities, and a marriage license.

But as I dug further into their situation, I discovered that there was a time, early in their marriage, that each day when he came home from work, they would spend thirty minutes to an hour talking about their day and how they thought and felt about it. It wasn't that he wasn't able to easily converse with her, it was that, over time, those conversations included less and less getting to know and understand each other and had become confrontations and attempts to change each other, leaving both feeling unaccepted. Eventually, the husband had no desire to listen to her when she said, "Can we talk?", because he knew that it was likely going to be about something she didn't like about him or what was wrong with their relationship. This dynamic is all too often what I see with couples who don't talk much or, when they do, usually end up arguing. There has got to be frequent and regular times when confrontation, talking about the relationship, and problem-solving are off-limits. This is why "date nights" and "dating for life" are important. If there is not more time spent in safe conversation, where none of those things are happening, there will be little or no productive conversation about things that need to be addressed concerning the two. That's because neither will feel accepted enough, by the other person, to feel safe enough to let their guards down. They will always approach discussions with their battle gear on and weapons in hand, a recipe for combative dialogue.

Quality time is as important as quantity time as well. Being there for the other person means a normal part of a daily routine. But some people can't sit down with each other, on a daily basis, because of schedules. However, I have seen great marriages where one or both spouses have a job that takes them out of town on a weekly basis. But they make an intentional effort to check in with each other, periodically, throughout the day, through phone calls or text messages. Many evenings end with one in bed at home and one in a hotel bed in another city. But, they are on the phone with each other, having that "goodnight" conversation that would be the same as the one they would be having if they were both home, a conversation that they both know is a safe time that they each can feel understood and accepted. I even recommend that couples have a designated "Safe" room in their home where they know they can sit with the other and that there will be no confrontation, problem-solving, or bringing up dissatisfaction with anything pertaining to the relationship. If you find that your spouse seems to avoid you when you want him or her to be there for you, it may be that they don't feel safe enough to do so. In that case, you will need to leave the deep end of the pool for a while and spend your time with them in the shallow end.

Commitment to Investing in the Relationship

I want to talk about South Dakota goat cheese farms for a while. Not interested? Me neither!

Okay, but what if I were to hack all your accounts and liquidate everything… your checking account, your savings, your retirement, your stocks, and so on, everything that could be liquidated for cash. The next day you received an email from me that read:

You may have noticed that you lost everything of monetary value last night. Take heart. You didn't. You still have it all in a stock portfolio. But here's the catch: That stock portfolio doesn't mature for five years. After those sixty months are up, you will be able to sell it for its value at market price. You could potentially be a very rich person in just five years!

The portfolio is made up of stocks in five promising goat cheese farms in South Dakota. Twenty percent of your investment has been placed in each farm. However, at any time the markets are open, you may move those percentages around. For example, tomorrow you could move all 100% into just one of those five stocks. The next day you could split that and put 50% in another farm and the other 50% in yet another.

Attached are the official certificate and the website where you can manage your portfolio.

Your account name: SDCheeseLover

Your password: GetYourGoat$

Overnight, your interest in South Dakota goat cheese farms would skyrocket! Why? Because you are now heavily invested in them! Instantly your life will change! You will now be choosing to check your stocks on the New York Stock Exchange. You'll eventually discover *Cheese Reporter* magazine (yes, that's a real thing) and start subscribing to it. Heck, you'll probably take a trip to South Dakota, just to see how these farms are doing!

Likewise, when two people are falling in limerence with each other, the same phenomenon happens. The two are spending almost all their extra resources on the relationship—their money, their time, and their energy. Then they get married, move in together, and, little by little, begin moving those investments into other stocks: Spending less and less money on dates and experiences together and more and more money on themselves; spending less and less energy on cultivating the relationship and more and more energy on their jobs, hobbies, or other relationships such as friends or family; spending less and less time planning on and being with each other and more and more time with....

And then one day they wake up and wonder why they have so little interest in the other person.

Just like finances, we gain interest by investing. And, just like the instant interest in goat cheese that comes from being heavily invested in it, you would be amazed at how interested you will become in your spouse if you pull a big investment out of something else in your life and put it back into your relationship!

For a lot of people, spending the money on a reputable marriage intensive is a sizeable hit to their pocketbook. I conduct about ten such intensives a year. Although I believe all marriages should make the invest-ment of attending at least one good intensive, most people tend to wait until their marriage gets very bad before they make such an investment. But, among those couples who attend ours, I frequently hear people tell me that things started getting better when they signed up and paid before the workshop even began. That is because they made a big investment.

Commitment to Growth

I went back for my graduate degree, in marriage and family therapy, about ten years into our marriage. In that city lived one of my old buddies from high school. Over that decade, or so, I had kept in touch with my old friend, but we had not really spent any time together. We'll call that old friend "Tim." So, I was really looking forward to reconnecting with Tim, and the fact that I wouldn't have to make a big effort to find a friend… I had a ready-made friend waiting for me there.

Tim and I played football together in high school. To be clearer, Tim played football. I was on the team, but I doubt that I contributed much. To earn your team letter, you had to play in at least sixteen quarters for the season. In our senior year, we went all the way through the playoffs to the state championship game. The team was so good that by the middle of the third quarter, we usually had enough of a lead that it was almost impos-sible for us to lose with me on the field (although sometimes I almost blew our lead). So, in my senior year, I played in exactly sixteen quarters, just enough to letter. Tim, on the other hand, was one of the best players on the team. He put everything he had into that playoff run, and it broke his heart when we got beat in the championship game.

As we were preparing to move there for my graduate degree, I asked

Tim to help me move our things into a storage unit until we could find an apartment. So, Tim and I spent the better part of a Saturday unloading the biggest U-Haul we could find. At first, I was excited to spend some time with Tim. There was a lot to catch up on with a decade now past. Later that evening, Joanna asked me if I had a good time hanging out with Tim again. But my reply was not a very positive one. There was more disappointment in my voice than excitement.

"I don't think I'm going to be hanging out with Tim much while we live here," I said. "All Tim wanted to talk about was going back in time, to December 1981, and the championship game. It was like hanging out with Uncle Rico all day" (another Napoleon Dynamite reference). "Tim doesn't seem to have grown up at all. I don't want to spend my free-buddy time with someone who is essentially still an eighteen-year old."

I see this same sentiment with many of the couples I work with, for example, a wife who continues to educate herself throughout the marriage, while her husband still spends most of his time playing video games or watching fifteen plus hours of sports a week. Or a husband who keeps up with current events and reads books to understand the world better, while his wife spends most of her free time on social media or binge-watching every episode of every season of every version of Crime Scene Specialist Investigation Victims Unit. I know these might sound like biased and sexist examples, but I see versions of these repeatedly. If your spouse is growing, and you're not, you're not committed. Could you imagine getting your annual review at work and telling your boss that you don't plan to get any better at your job in the future and expecting her to accept that?

Another reason that commitment to growth is important is because love is not natural. We don't naturally know how to love well. To love means to get better at loving and learn how to love better and better. Love is dynamic, it's not stagnant. You are either getting better at loving or getting worse at loving. An eighteen-year old is expected to love like an eighteen-year old. But a thirty-five-year old who loves like an eighteen-year old is just immature.

Commitment to Supportive Social Structures

In our early years of marriage, like most couples, we recognized that we needed couple friends. We somehow understood that it is important to transition from just having his friends and her friends toward more "our friends." As we met other married couples, however, who seemed to have similar values to ours, we noticed a pattern: When Joanna clicked with the wife of a newly met couple, I didn't seem to feel much of a connection with the husband. And, when I found a husband I enjoyed being around, Joanna didn't feel the same about the wife.

If you have experienced the same thing, now you know you're not alone. Actually, this phenomenon is more common that not. The biggest reason is simple mathematics. What percentage of people that you meet, on a daily basis, do you think you could easily become close friends with? And how many of those do you think having a friendship with would help you become a better person? I don't know about you, but, for me, that answer would be a mayyybeee one percent. That answer might indicate the source of many of my issues, but, for argument's sake, let's say for you it's ten percent. Now, many people think that finding a close friend-couple should only be double the difficulty, since there are now two of us. So that figure would now become five percent. However, there are less people that are part of a couple than there are individual people in general, so that figure would come down to at least four percent. But here's where so many get the math wrong. It's actually exponentially more difficult to find a couple friend, not just twice as difficult. Husband of couple A must feel a connection with both the husband and wife of couple B. Wife of couple B must connect with both spouses of couple A and so on. These tables should help to illustrate the differences in likelihood.

Requirements for 2 People to Connect as Close Friends

Persons A and B feel connected to each other

Requirements for 2 Couples to Connect as Close Friends

Husband of couple A feels connected to husband of couple B
Husband of couple A feels connected to wife of couple B
Wife of couple A feels connected to wife of couple B
Wife of couple A feels connected to husband of couple B
Husband of couple B feels connected to husband of couple A
Husband of couple B feels connected to wife of couple A
Wife of couple B feels connected to wife of couple A
Wife of couple B feels connected to husband of couple A

Now, here's where my mathematical skills begin to run afoul, so let's just say that it is eight hundred percent easier to find a single close friend than to find a close friend-couple.

So, what do you do? Well, there are a few websites that offer to help you find couple friends, for a fee of course. But, even if you use those services, like Internet dating, you won't truly know if you connect well until you spend some time together. More commonly, we meet our couple friends in social settings that are important to us: church, work, neighborhoods, family, and so on. It's just not likely that you're all going to feel an instant eight-way connection right off the bat. What is more important, though, is that they are *supportive* friends. In other words, being around them makes your own marriage better. There is no middle ground here. The people in your life will play one of two roles. They will either make your marriage better, or they will make it worse. They can't be neutral, even if they try. So, find people who care as much about your marriage as they care about you as an individual because, the thing is, if they truly care about you, then they must care about the most important human relationship in your life!

Almost all our couple friends (Joanna's and mine) are people that one of us didn't connect well with at first. But we chose to nurture those relationships because we knew they truly cared about us as a couple and valued the things and ideas that we most valued in life. Although some of them are nothing like me, because they intentionally support and accept us, over the years they have become deep, lifelong friends. We take vacations together. Our children call them "aunt" and "uncle." They are the ones who are truly there when other so-called friends have moved on from our lives. Those friendships didn't develop naturally. They developed intentionally.

Family is also typically part of one's social structure, although we don't usually choose family to be a part of it. But, some people would do well to move certain family members toward the outer edges of their social circles. I have dealt with many couples who have a parent or sibling that is severely affecting their marriage in a negative way. I have advised many of these people to have a serious talk with that family member that goes something like this:

Dad, I know you have my best interests at heart, but your actions are actually making matters worse. My spouse is my most important human relationship, and you will either be a part of reinforcing my marriage for the better, or you will make things worse. So, unless you start being on "our" side instead of just "my" side, I can't be around you. I love you, but I need to love my spouse more!

By the way, this is a conversation that needs to start with the spouse that is a member of the family member involved. It goes back to the core—acceptance. How accepted can one possibly feel if their mate chooses family over spouse? I have seen many marriages have a huge turnaround, for the better, simply because one spouse stood up for the other, in front of their own family.

Commitment to Having No Alternatives

The conquering of indigenous people, in the Americas, was made up of many horrible atrocities on the part of mostly European people and their descendants. One of these famous conquerors was a Spaniard by the name of Hernán Cortés. In fact, he and his armies were referred to as conquerors or "Conquistadors." There are many stories that attempt to explain why so few Spaniards were able to conquer so many indigenous people. The most famous one was when he had his ships destroyed at the port of what is now Veracruz, Mexico. From there he and his army of less than 700 went on to eventually take over the entire Aztec Nation, believed to be more than a million people. This "burning of the ships" made it so that there was no way to escape, should they encounter forces that might drive them back into the sea. With no alternative except to wholeheartedly take part in his plan to conquer the Aztecs, Cortés' army not only fought differently, the day-to-day routines of traveling to interior Mexico, and preparing for battles, brought on different attitudes among the men, which they would not have had if there was an escape route or alternative plan.

Likewise, a marriage is almost certainly doomed to failure if either or both spouses have a backup plan. If there is an alternative to staying married when times are tough, that alternative will at least be considered. Once one spouse begins considering the alternative, that option will become more and more desirable, causing the relationship to become less and less stable. It's like the eighteen-year old in the last semester of high school. Once he sees that he can slack off and still graduate, senioritis sets in and what was once a 3.8 GPA ends up a 2.5.

Some people have no alternative plans to being married to their spouse, yet they continually put the other on what I call "relationship probation." They do this because they believe that they will be happier if the other spouse would only act differently. We've already talked about how this mindset makes people *less* happy, but what those with this mindset don't realize is that it actually makes the relationship less stable as well. In their unhappiness, they attempt to coerce the other to being different by making it seem as if they are not "all in." This *relationship probation* can take many forms:

Threatening divorce or separation
Withholding affection
Withholding love
Withholding acceptance
Withholding sex or conversation

These are some of the more common examples I encounter.

So why do people do these things if they have no real intention of ending the marriage? Well, it's because they tend to work… at first. They are nothing more than idle threats that, early on, seem to get others' attention. However, as time goes on, the threats must increase in intensity for them to be as effective. Like heroin, you must keep upping the dose to get the same results. And, like heroin, the eventual outcome is death of the marriage. Going back to the basis of this book, it portrays a sense of unacceptance because the other spouse continually feels less and less like they will ever be off probation… ever be accepted.

A few years ago, I worked with a couple who had been married for over thirty years and had been separated seventeen times in those thirty years. The first separation came about just before the wedding. The limerence had worn off, and the wife began to see some things about her future husband that she didn't think she could live with. So, after the invitations had already gone out, she notified him that the wedding was off. He begged and pleaded with her, telling her that he would change, so she decided to go ahead and marry him. A few short months into the marriage came separation number two. He had changed some of the things she wanted him to change. Some of those changes didn't last long, though. So, the wife, noticing how it got his attention the first time, told him to move out. A few days later, he called her begging to come home and promising more change. The third separation came about a year later. Again, some changes had occurred, some changes reverted back to the old ways, and some of the changes she had hoped for didn't occur at all. Each subsequent separation got longer as the time between got shorter.

Before I found out about all these separations, I asked her why she had come to me. Her reply was that their marriage had never been a good one, from day one. That's when I had her walk back through time with me as she told me about the first separation, before the wedding, and then about five or six of the subsequent separations. The story of each separation was basically the same thing, over and over again.

"So, your marriage has always been on probation!", I exclaimed.

"What do you mean?", she asked.

"Well, your husband has never felt like you accept him. You've had him on probation for over thirty years. It's a wonder your marriage lasted this long. A marriage on probation will never be a good marriage. It lacks the central ingredient: acceptance!"

Building Relational Wealth vs. Avoiding Relational Bankruptcy

BUILDING RELATIONAL WEALTH VS. AVOIDING RELATIONAL BANKRUPTCY

Early in my marriage, when things weren't going so well and I was investing less and less on our relationship, Joanna and I had a joint checking account. This was back in the 1980s and checks were used for far more things than they are today. We didn't have the Internet, so all our bills were paid by sending a check in the mail. When we bought groceries, we paid by check. There was no such thing as debit cards, only credit cards that charged extra fees and rates when used. Also, unlike the checkbooks of today, there was no carbon copy backup. Instead, there was a ledger, at the front of the checkbook. Each time you wrote a check, you were expected to record the check number, date, entity to which the check was written, and the amount of the check. Finally, you were supposed to balance your checkbook to reflect the new amount you now had in your account after writing the check.[1]

Many times, I would be standing in the checkout line at the grocery

---

[1] I just sent the same text to each of my three adult children, ages twenty-nine, twenty-six, and twenty-two, asking them if they owned a checkbook. Only the oldest replied that she did. She's been married for six years and owns a house with her husband. So, this analogy might not relate well to some of the younger readers.

store, writing out my check, and noticing that there were several people waiting impatiently in line behind me. So, I would tell myself that I would fill out the register as soon as I got in my vehicle, so as to speed the line along and ease the frustration of my fellow shoppers. Most of the time, however, by the time I had gotten into my vehicle, my mind was on something else and I forgot to record the check. A day or two later, I would write another check based on what the balance was before I wrote that check at the grocery store. But there were not enough funds to cover that check. Again, this was before the Internet or banking apps on smartphones that let us know what our balance is. I wouldn't find out that I had written a hot check until about a week later when I received a snail mail letter from the bank, informing me that, not only is my balance in the negative, they have also added an overdraft charge of $20.

This happened five or six times before my bank got fed up and finally sent me a letter saying they were closing our account. What was I going to do without a checking account? I really needed a checking account! So, I drove to the bank and begged them to reopen my account. The begging didn't work. However, they said I could open a *different* checking account with five hundred dollars. With this new account, they would honor a check if it put the balance below five hundred dollars, but they would still apply a service fee. They told me that the point of a bank account was to build wealth, not just pay bills.

In those days I was treating my relationship to Joanna with the same mindset I had for my checking account. I thought that as long as I don't go below the zero line, then I'm being a good steward with my money. Like my checking account, my goal was to avoid bankruptcy. I wasn't thinking about building wealth. As long as Joanna wasn't mad or frustrated with me, I thought to myself, *then I'm being a good husband!*. If I had twenty-five "relational dollars" in the account, I'm good to go! I wasn't thinking about increasing that balance, more and more over time, so that we would have a buffer for when I really screwed up. Like my checking account, I had to work extra hard, writing hot checks and then having to pay to get myself out of the hole.

This has a lot to do with why many people say that marriage is hard work. They're just trying to stay out of trouble instead of continually investing in the relationship and building wealth. Every little hurtful word, every little mistake, whether intended or not, becomes a deficit that puts the relationship in the hole. They must work harder and harder in order to make up for those overdraft charges that also come with relationships. You can easily spot these people. They're continually attempting to avoid being in the proverbial "Doghouse" and will check in now and then with an "Are we good?", just making sure that they have a few pennies above the zero line.

On the other hand, you can spot a spouse who has been building relational wealth. They can say something rude or sarcastic to their husband or wife, and it just rolls off like water on a dragon's butt (or is it a duck's back, I don't remember). Even when big things happen, like losing a job or saying something very hurtful, it doesn't stress the relationship as much because there's a large balance in the relational account that covers the damages. People who build relational wealth tend to have marriages that are much more stable and much less work. These are the people who will tell you that being married is much less work than being single.

It's important to understand that building relational wealth takes time. With an actual checking account, you can make a hundred-thousand-dollar deposit, but the banker doesn't get excited about it if you turn around and write someone a check for the same amount. Relational accounts operate much the same way. Even if you have a history of never dipping below the zero line, your spouse isn't going to feel very secure in the relationship if every time you make a big deposit you withdraw it the next day. In fact, if that sort of behavior becomes the norm, those big deposits will become more and more suspect to your spouse. They will begin to wonder what your ulterior motives are for doing so. It will take some time of building relational wealth before she or he begins to trust that you are truly investing in the relationship, not just setting them up for disappointment.

It is important to distinguish between a *relational account* and the idea of "keeping score." *Keeping score* is when I consciously keep track of the relational deposits and withdrawals of my mate, and likely includes letting her know when I think she has done less than me for the relationship. This is a recipe for disaster!

A relational account, on the other hand, is just that subconscious ledger that each spouse carries around in their head, based on their own perception of how each is contributing to the relationship. If we are striving toward truly loving our mate, we must recognize that we have that subconscious ledger and that it is based on our *perceptions*, not all the facts. So, we must remind ourselves that we tend to see our own deposits as larger than they are and our mate's withdrawals as larger than they are. I tell my clients: "Start every day by ripping up your own ledger and coming up with a way that you can make a deposit in your mate's account that day."

Finally, it is important to understand that you each deal in your own relational currency. What may seem like a deposit to you may be a withdrawal to your spouse.

Early in our marriage, I would try to get myself out of the "Doghouse" by picking up a dozen roses on the way home from work. Joanna was gracious when I made this effort, but she didn't seem to be as pleased as I thought she should be. It was a few years before I found out why:

1. She didn't like roses.
2. The reason I was making the relational deposit in the first place was because the day before we had received a letter from the bank stating that I had written a bad check and we now had to pay an additional service charge.

This attempt at making a deposit was actually a withdrawal. Later I learned that had I just come home and cleaned the toilets, it would have made a huge deposit.

We Don't Have a Power Struggle?

We Don't Have a
Power Struggle?

How often have you had some version of the following conversation?

> Spouse 1: "Are you hungry?"
> Spouse 2: "I could eat something."
> Spouse 1: "Yeah, I'm getting hungry too!"
> Spouse 2: "So, what do you feel like?"
> Spouse 1: "What do you feel like?"
> Spouse 2: "I don't really care, what do you feel like?"
> Spouse 1: "I could eat just about anything. What sounds good to you?"
> Spouse 2: "You pick. I'm good with anything."
> Spouse 1: "Same here, what sounds good to you?"

...

My experience is that this is at least a weekly conversation between spouses. What if I told you that it is a power struggle?

You would likely tell me, "No! I'm attempting to relinquish power... let my spouse decide."

That may be true in some cases. However, in most cases, that's only a piece of what's happening. Usually, when one spouse says something like, "You pick," they are attempting to be nice. But if we could get inside their heads and see what they are *really* thinking, it would sound something like this:

"Sweetheart, I really, really want you to pick out a place for us to eat and that *I* want to eat at."

Still don't believe me? Let's play this scenario out a little further. Let's say the back-and-forth between spouse 1 and spouse 2 goes on a little further, and it looks something like this:

Spouse 2: "Okay. If you insist. I'll pick. Let's go to McDonald's drive-up window and each pick three things off the value menu and then take it home and watch the game."

Spouse 1: "Well, I wasn't thinking about getting fast food, I was thinking about something healthy where we could sit down, talk, and catch up on each other's day."

Spouse 2: "Well, that's not what you said. You told me to pick, so I picked. It didn't matter much to me. I gave you the opportunity to pick, more than once, but you told me to pick, so I picked."

Joanna and I have had hundreds, if not thousands, of these conversations. When our children were younger, before we took parenting classes and thought that we would instinctively know how to parent well, the conversation would pick up, from there, something like this:

Spouse 2: "So, since you told me to pick, I picked. We're going to McDonald's! Everyone, start figuring out what you want before we get there so we don't hold up the line!"

Spouse 1: "Well kids, I guess your dad doesn't really care about your health or his family. Apparently, all he cares about is filling his tummy and watching the game!"

If we look what is behind that stance that spouse number 2 has taken, we will probably surmise something that makes us believe the following:

Spouse 2 wants to eat cheap.
Spouse 2 wants to eat fast.
Spouse 2 wants to watch the game.

Spouse 2 is not concerned with having a healthy meal.

Spouse 2 wants to enjoy family time by watching his team together.

But what if the tables were turned? What if, earlier in the conversation, it went something like this?

Spouse 1: "Okay, I'll pick. Let's go eat at *De Bon Gout.*"

Before we go any further, I'm sure there is a restaurant, somewhere out there, named *De Bon Gout.* If so, and your food is good, at reasonable prices, please forgive me! That being said, I simply Googled "French for Tasty" and that's what I got. So, as far as I'm concerned, it's not a real restaurant. For the purposes of this analogy, *De Bon Gout* is a fancy restaurant. It is gourmet food, served in gourmet portions (otherwise known as tiny portions), at gourmet prices (otherwise known as expensive), on a gourmet clock (otherwise known as two or more hours, you'll miss the game).

Now, if we were to guess at what Spouse 1 wants, we might surmise the following:

Spouse 1 wants to have a meal that involves interaction among the family.

Spouse 1 wants to eat tasty food.

Spouse 1 wants to eat healthy food.

Spouse 1 wants the meal, in and of itself, to be a positive experience.

Spouse 1 sees the extra cost, of time and money, as an investment in the family.

Now, let's set all of this aside for the moment and talk about *power dynamics.*

Earlier in our marriage, before I got my degree in marriage and family therapy, my thinking was that a marriage could not resemble a democracy because it is only made up of two people. Every decision that affects both spouses is either going to end up as one that is unanimous or split. So, in the case of split decisions, one person needs to be the tiebreaker.

Based on the cultural norms I grew up with, I believed that tiebreaker was the husband.

But when you look at the dynamics that occur when two people want different things—the dynamics of power—eventually, if power is not being shared, one person will step into the *overt* power position, and then the other will slip into the *covert* power position. The overt power is the power position that is obvious. It's usually the person that is talking the loudest, or making demands, or putting his proverbial "foot down." The covert power, on the other hand, is just like it sounds. It's covert. It's less obvious and detectable. What is extremely important to understand, however, is that the covert power is just as powerful as the overt power and, in some instances, can be even more powerful!

In the first scenario, where Spouse 2 ends up making the decision to eat McDonald's, he has taken a stand and stepped firmly into the overt power position. But notice what Spouse 1 says, once she has realized that she will now struggle from the covert power position:

Spouse 1: "Well kids, I guess your dad doesn't really care about your health or his family. Apparently, all he cares about is filling his tummy and watching the game!"

For the purposes of comparing and contrasting, let's say that things went the other way, that Spouse 1 took on the overt power position and said something like, "Okay, I'll pick. We're going to *De Bon Gout!*" In this scenario, Spouse 1 has begun to claim the overt power position. Let's see how this plays out:

Spouse 2: "Hold on a minute! This ain't Valentine's Day! I thought we were just going to get some food for the family, not watch our kids waste forty bucks each on food they won't even eat!"

Spouse 1: "You said you didn't care where we ate. You told me to choose. You insisted I choose! I wanted you to choose but you wouldn't. You told me to choose and you said you'd be fine with anything. Well, not only does *De Bon Gout* fall under the category of *anything*, it specifically falls under the subset of *anything known as restaurants*! You told me to pick. I picked. We're going to *De Bon Gout*!"

Spouse 1 has now inserted herself firmly into the overt position. Let's see what Spouse 2 does:

Spouse 2: "Well kids, it looks like we're not going to be able to pay the electricity bill this month because mom has to eat at Ow, Bone Pain!"

Spouse 1: "No, we're going to *De Bon Gout*, not *Au Bon Pain*, that's in the airport."

Spouse 2: "Bone gout, bone pain, they both sound more like a health problem than a place to eat. I get bone gout just thinking that most of what I'm paying for is to look at the expensive art on the wall. We could eat at McDonald's *and* go to an art museum for less than half the cost and still be done thirty minutes faster!"

Or sometimes, the covert power can be even more powerful by saying nothing at all. It can just silently stare out the car window with a look that let's the whole family know that the other spouse will pay, and we're not talking just for the meal. Whether they are dining at De Bon Gout or slamming down junk food in front of the TV, the silence ruins the day for everyone, and the kids can't wait until the meal is over so they can get away from the tension. Everybody loses, even the spouse that seemed to get his or her way, when power isn't being shared.

Most couples go through a period in their marriage when more and more issues end up being power struggles where nobody really wins. At first, the two usually have more energy and willingness to come to a mutual agreement. He's found an apartment that's close to his job and will give him more time at home with her and the baby that's on the way. She's found one that's close to her parent's, and they're going to have to rely a lot on her parents for childcare. So, they compromise and find another one that's halfway between.

But as time goes on, they begin to encounter issues that seem less negotiable. She wants the children to attend public school. He wants them to attend private school and believes his reasoning on the matter is much more sound than hers, not to mention that he believes his reasoning is a moral issue. One day he puts his foot down and exclaims, "Our kids are getting a private education and that's final!" He has stepped firmly into the overt power position, so she must now take on the covert power. And here's another way the covert power position can be so powerful: she may decide to lose this one, in order to win another one that means even more to her.

"Well, if you're going to get to win that one then I'm going to declare that, from now on, we will be attending my parent's church!"

Although he doesn't really like her parent's church, he sees that he won the first one, so it's only fair. They've each claimed an important "mountain" in their relationship and stuck a proverbial flag in it, marking it as their own territory. But then, they begin to survey that territory and realize that there are other important issues that they don't see eye to eye on. So begins the race to claim territory. He sticks a flag on the hill of *finances*. She plants one firmly on the hill of *parenting*. So, he races to plant his flag on the smaller hill of where they will build their first house, while she scrambles to claim a ranch style over his preferred two story. Before long, every issue in their relationship either has a "hers" or "his" flag stuck in it, down to the smallest ant hill. So, every time they encounter these issues, there is an automatic atmosphere of war. One of us is going to lose and one of us is going to win.

There is a couple that is very close to us who would try to solve these issues quickly by playing "rock/paper/scissors." Even though it seemed, at first, that issues were being solved with this method, most of them really weren't. Sure, it might work for matters of less importance such as whether to watch *Seinfeld* or *Friends*, but the bigger issues were not really solved. If one believed they should use their savings on a vacation, while the other believed it should go toward buying a more dependable vehicle, the one who lost on rock/paper/scissors is not likely to let it go... they have simply fallen into the covert power position. Even though he agreed to go on the vacation, he at least will likely spoil some of the vacation by constantly reminding her that if her car breaks down, she will now have to take the bus to work. Power hasn't been truly shared and both end up losing.

Now, think about each of these issues as a roundtable, about three feet in diameter. Imagine that each of these tables has as many pennies as you could place on it, just one-penny deep. I could stop right here and take about ten minutes to do the math, with the help of the Internet of course, but I think it's safe to say that there would be hundreds of pennies on each table. Each of those pennies represents a different solution to the issue. This is simply for argument's sake. However, there is an infinite amount of solutions to most any issue. When someone tells me they've tried *everything*, in attempts to solve an issue, I remind them that's impossible. There's always another thing that has yet to be tried.

As couples begin to struggle over more and more issues, the attempts to claim territory play out with each person choosing the penny that to him or her looks like the best solution. One puts a thumb firmly on his favorite penny, while the other puts a thumb on her favorite. They now see these two pennies as the only potential solutions. So, to simplify matters, they use the other hand to rake off all the other pennies onto the floor. After a while, as they look around the room of tables, each one now only has two pennies on it. All the other possible solutions are soon forgotten. There's now only your way or mine. Every issue becomes a power struggle, and eventually the two can't talk about much at all without it feeling like a battle.

The solution starts with that penny under *your* thumb! It's gotta go! It won't work anyway. Even if that penny wins the battle and gets chosen, remember, the covert power will sabotage it.

People often ask me to recommend a parenting class. Joanna and I took five parenting classes. The first one we took three times. Because we waited until our oldest child was about eight years old, and we had become so entrenched in some bad parenting practices, we had to go back a year later and take it again, and again a year after that. We've read books on parenting and gone to parenting seminars as well. Remember, good parenting doesn't come naturally, so you'll save a lot of time, money, and heartache by starting before they're born!

Even then, how do you decide which one to take? Start with doing your research! Which ones have the best reputations and are widely used? My opinion shouldn't matter much. I think you should take more than one so that you have balancing perspectives. But even if I told you my favorite, it's not going to work well for you if your spouse isn't fully on board. The best parenting class for you may be way down my list, but it's the one in which you are both fully in agreement to take.

So, on the table that is labeled "Our First Parenting Class," if you each have a penny on that table, your first step is to pick yours up and throw it as far as you can away from the table, even if your spouse doesn't do the same with hers or his. That bears repeating. You've got to remove your penny, even if your significant other has no intention of removing theirs. Simply removing yours will at least help your spouse to ease their thumb pressure and maybe even start looking on the floor for other optional pennies.

Your next step is to scan the floor to find the penny that would most satisfy both of your concerns. You may not get it right on the first or second try. Hang in there. The very process of looking for, and offering up, a possible mutually satisfying solution will, in and of itself, help your spouse feel more and more like you are letting go of some power, helping them to feel less desperate to cling to theirs. As you get better at finding that mutually satisfying solution, and offering it to your spouse, you will notice that matters begin to be solved much more quickly, not to mention your feelings toward each other will improve vastly.

When Joanna and I were at the height of our power struggle years and getting ready to go somewhere that mattered to her, I would occasionally put on an outfit that I knew she wouldn't like. As this stubbornness progressed, she became much more opinionated about how I dressed. Then we went to a marriage seminar where they told us that we should strive to make *all* our decisions based on consideration for our spouse and that both of us should feel positive about those decisions. So, I began to apply that concept. When we were getting ready to go out, I would go into the closet and look for something I thought she would be pleased to see me wear. Then I would show it to her and ask her what she thought. At first, she often told me that I was way off the mark. Much of that was due to the fact that she was accustomed to me flaunting my defiance of her wishes. But as time went on, and she knew I was considering her, it became less and less important to her what I wore. There was a lot more grace given for the times I picked out a shirt that didn't at all go with the pants I'd selected. These days, I know that I'm wearing something that clashes like ketchup and chocolate when she says, "Why don't you FaceTime one of the girls and get their opinion."

The fact of the matter is that we have *more* influence (power) when we share power. Conversely, we lose power the more we attempt to be in control. Healthy growing marriages are ones in which both spouses make all their decisions based on the idea that the decision will be one that they can both feel good about.

By the way, making a unilateral decision and then attempting to get your spouse to agree with it is the opposite of what we're talking about. That's simply coercion and it will backfire in the long run. Even if you have an idea that you believe is the best choice, and you present it to your spouse in a manner that sends the signal that you've already made up your mind, that idea will not end up being the best idea.

A friend of mine shared a story with me that makes this point even clearer. His name is Phil. Phil is the CEO and co-founder of a very successful company that has offices all over the world. If you met Phil at the grocery store, you wouldn't know he has a lot of money. He doesn't dress like it, his car doesn't reflect it, and, most importantly, his demeanor wouldn't tell you anything other than he is a humble and caring husband and father. I hadn't seen Phil for several years until recently. We were eating lunch together, and I did my best to retell this story back to him to see how badly I had twisted it over the years. I tell this story at least once a month, usually to audiences attending one of our seminars, so I wanted to make sure I was telling it with integrity. After reciting it back to Phil, all he said was something like, "That was pretty close." He didn't correct me on any of the details so here we go.

When Phil and his partner started their company, they believed that their plan would be hugely successful, that in no time they would have hundreds or thousands of employees, with offices all over the world. However, some years later they came to the conclusion that they should hire a consultant because they had not yet grown to anywhere close to their expectations. Hopefully this consultant would help them figure out what they were doing wrong. After the consultant had spent some time studying their company and how they operated, he came back with a recommendation.

He explained to them that their business plan was great, no problem there. The problem was *how* they carried out that plan. Up until that time, when Phil and his partner had a new idea for the company to implement, they would call in the top-level management, present to them their plan, and then direct them to carry it out. Each top-level manager would then meet with her managers and present the new initiative and charge them with carrying it out. Finally, those managers would then meet with all the employees under them, giving them their new "marching orders." That was how things were being done before the consultant stepped in. Then he explained what he believed they should be doing differently.

From now on, when the two of you have an idea to implement, call in your top-level managers. Instead of telling them what they are supposed to do, simply present your idea as just that... and idea that you are considering. Then ask for their input and critique. If all of you come to a consensus, then you're ready for step 2. Keep in mind that the consensus may end up looking very different from your original idea.

For step 2, once consensus has been reached, have the top-level managers take this new idea to each of their mid-level managers and go through the same process, presenting it as an idea, not a directive, getting their input and critique, and then arriving at a consensus before taking it down the chain to the next level of employees. If consensus can't be reached, kick it back up the chain to the executives. Step 3 is to have all the mid-level managers then do the same with the remainder of employees under their supervision, until everyone in the company has had input in the decision.

When Phil was telling me this story for the first time, at this point I thought to myself, "But that would be terribly inefficient. Not to mention, a really good plan could easily get watered down into a mediocre plan or worse." That's when Phil explained further.

He and his partner decided to give a try; although they had some strong reservations about the idea, nothing else seemed to be working. Within a short time, though, things started picking up. Employee satisfaction began to rise. Productivity was up. They were gaining more clients and making more money. Now, they were doing so well that they had to hire more and more employees in order to keep up with the demand of their services.

Why? Because now, *all* the employees felt like they had a say in their job. They had influence on decisions that were made that affected their own jobs. They now had power. The result was that they were much more willing to go along with the decisions being made, because they were a part of making those decisions. The consultant recognized that the best idea is actually a bad idea if it is being pushed upon the employees without their buy-in. On the other hand, when we believe we have had a say in coming up with a plan, we are much more likely to enthusiastically be a part of carrying out that plan. If we believe we are being coerced to simply carry out someone else's plan, even if it's a great plan, we will at least drag our feet, if not sabotage it, all together.

Let's revisit the restaurant scenario one last time.

There is a restaurant Joanna and I both like. We'll call it "Maria's." If it were a typical work day and we were going to eat lunch alone, neither of us would likely pick Maria's. Instead, we would probably choose a restaurant that we personally like but our spouse doesn't care much for. However, Maria's is a great "penny on the floor" for us. It has tasty and healthy food. The prices are very reasonable. The atmosphere is pleasant and clean. The staff is friendly and professional. And, they get you your food amazingly quick.

If instead of saying, "Joanna, where would you like to eat?" I had said something like, "How do you feel about eating at Maria's?" nine times out of ten, Joanna is going to say something like, "Sounds great!"

It's not at the top of her personal list. It's not at the top of my personal list. It's at the top of *our* list! The one time out of ten? Joanna would say something like, "I'm good with Maria's or we could eat at *The Grill*. We haven't been there in a while."

The Grill isn't even in Joanna's top ten. But she knows it's in my top five. Because she knows I'm sharing power with her, she is feeling accepted and loved. She wants to return the sentiment.

MARRIAGE HELP
DOESN'T

Marriage Help
Doesn't

Let's say your marriage is struggling a bit. You don't necessarily dislike your spouse, but you're not exactly thrilled about them either. One day you see an advertisement that a famous marriage guru is coming to town to speak on the subject: *How to Reignite Your Marriage.*

"That's exactly what we need," you think to yourself. "I'm going to get us tickets!" So, you get online and make your purchase. You're so excited to tell your spouse. But, for some reason, they don't seem very thrilled, although they agree to go. Why doesn't he or she share your enthusiasm? Because, they believe that you are hoping it will change *them* more than it will *yourself.*

A month later you are sitting in the audience with your spouse. Not only is the speaker funny and engaging, she is presenting a lot of great tools. She tells the audience that you should never blame your own feelings on your spouse, something your spouse often does to you. She tells the audience that you should give respect to your spouse, even when they aren't acting respectably, something you need to get better about doing. You make a mental note to show more respect. You make an *actual* note, in the margin of your handout: *don't blame your feelings on your spouse!* You're feeling really great about coming to this event. You've learned some things that will help you. But, most importantly, your spouse heard some things that should really, really help him or her be a better spouse. You have more hope for your marriage!

A week later, you have an argument…

Spouse: "This is the second time, since we went to that marriage event, that you made me feel disrespected!"

You: "Well, this is at least the third time, since we went to that event, that you blamed your feelings on me!"

We can all see where this is going, so I won't bore you with the entire dialogue. At the end of the argument, things now seem to be worse than before the event, creating an even greater sense that there is something fundamentally wrong with the relationship. But as my good friend Tim Russo likes to say: "There's nothing wrong with your marriage!"

You see, a relationship is not a real thing. You can't drop your relationship off at my office and hear me say something like, "Come back in six weeks to pick up your relationship. I should have it running just fine." A relationship is simply what we label the dynamics of how two individuals interact with each other. Let's look at it in another way,

The other day I had a couple in my office. I had been assigning them to have at least five "Us Time" discussions per week. "Us Time" is what I used to call those conversations that happen in the shallow end of the relationship pool. You talk about more of the superficial things in life. Neither is allowed to bring up situations they think need to be addressed. Neither is allowed to confront the other about anything. And, neither is allowed to bring up any issues about their marriage or relationship. The idea here is to create an atmosphere where both feel safer to be vulnerable with each other. So, I usually assign the topic: *this is what it was like to be me today*. I encourage them to talk about the things that are going on in their daily life that don't directly involve the interaction (relationship) between the two of them. But I missed one key element. This couple worked together. They ran a business together. They were interacting with each other all day! It felt awkward to them because they already knew about everything the other was telling them.

After a few weeks, the wife said, "When will we get to start talking about *Us*?"

"What do you mean by that?", I asked. "What does *talking about Us* look like to you?"

"You know," she replied, "Our stuff. Our issues. Our problems with each other."

I had a good notion that's what she meant. So, I jumped on the opportunity.

"There is no *Us*! There are only two individuals relating to each other. *Us* doesn't have a problem because *Us* does not exist. You exist and your husband exists. You have problems in the way you relate to him, and he has problems in the way he relates to you. When you tell your husband that you want to talk about *Us*, which one of those people's problems is he likely thinking you want to address? His, of course! So, why would he want to go to the deep end with you if he knows that you're going to talk about what's wrong with him? Nobody wants to be in over their head with someone they don't feel safe with, someone who is going to point out that they are not acceptable."

This is why most approaches to helping marriages fail in the long run, not because they are lacking in good information but, rather, because the good information tends to get applied to "Us" rather than to "Me." When we attempt to apply it to "Us," we are actually applying it to the other person, attempting to change them. Remember, attempts to change someone are clear messages of unacceptance. Not to mention, you can't change someone else anyway.

We could power the entire world's energy needs if we could simply harness the wasted energy that goes into trying to change others. We could solve the world's economic dilemmas if we could redistribute the resources wasted on attempting to change our spouses. We could have weeks of extra free time, each year, if we would save the time that is wasted on trying to get our husband or wife to be different! Those are all wasted resources because they are spent on something we can't accomplish—changing someone else.

When we try to change someone else, we are powerless, not to mention that we make matters worse because they feel less accepted. But there is power to be found when we change ourselves!

You see, a relationship, although not a tangible thing, is a system. And, one rule of *all* systems is that, if one part of the system changes, the whole system changes. In other words, if I get better at being a spouse, my marriage can't help but get better, regardless of whether my spouse gets better. This truth is at the core of why our intensives are so much more effective than traditional methods of helping marriages. Without a grasp of this truth, we are attempting to solve our problems with a mindset that not only leaves us powerless, but also will eventually destroy the foundation of what brought the two together in the first place—the belief that they were each accepted by the other.

When a wife asks me, "How do I get my husband to stop... (fill in the blank with what you would like your mate to stop doing)", my answer is "You can't."

When a husband asks me, "What do I do to get my wife to... (fill in the blank with something you wish your spouse would do differently)", my answer is "You don't."

"What could *you* do differently?", I ask.

"Oh, I've tried everything," they will often answer. "Nothing seems to get them to change!"

There are two things wrong here: First, they are still talking about trying to change their spouse. You can't. Second, you can *never* try *everything*. There's always another way to approach any issue. Want to feel less depressed? Want to feel less anxious? Want to experience more peace and joy? Want to have better relationships with everyone, especially your mate? Free yourself from trying to change people!

From now on, I am changing the term "Us Time" to "You and Me Time."

PERPETUAL FORGIVENESS

Perpetual Forgiveness

One of the biggest movie hits of 1970 was a film called *Love Story*. The famous line of that movie is "Love means not ever having to say you're sorry." As if two people love each other, they're never going to hurt each other or wrong one another. Hogwash! We're humans! We're going to mess up! Forgiveness is going to be a crucial piece of any good relationship, much more so with a lifelong mate.

For most people that's a given. But, even for those couples who have pronounced forgiveness toward their spouse for something that may have happened five years ago, there is still often a sense that forgiveness wasn't complete, by both the offended and the person who did the deed. In the case of extramarital affairs, we often see some version of the following:

Wife: *I forgave him years ago but there still seems to be something left undone. I don't trust him, and it's like it's all just been swept under the rug.*

Husband: *I know I messed up. I asked her to forgive me. She said she forgave me. But it's like she hasn't moved on. I don't know how you can say you forgave someone, but you keep bringing it up. Holding it over my head.*

It doesn't have to be sexual infidelity. It could be almost anything: lying, a hurtful word, a threat, a major purchase without including the other, and so on; whatever is done, or failed to be done, that damages the relationship, must go through the process of forgiveness. But it must be understood that forgiveness is a *process*.

Many people consider forgiveness as an exchange of phrases:

Do you forgive me?
Yes, I forgive you!

While those two phrases are important, they are only a small part of a much bigger process. Just saying a simple phrase doesn't make one forget. A simple phrase doesn't transform a heart. A simple phrase doesn't repair the damage done. A simple phrase doesn't rebuild trust. There must be so much more. And, it might take days, months, or even years. But the sooner both parties wade into that process, the sooner those things will be accomplished. The more we avoid the process, the slower complete forgiveness occurs, and the more damage is done. We aren't God. As humans, we can choose to *forgive*, but we can't choose to *forget*. The longer we avoid the process, the more the event stays at the forefront of our memory.

When we do something to wrong another human being, whether big or small, it creates consequences. Those consequences each create their own set of consequences, which then create still further consequences. The event can't be understood in isolation. Its results ripple out in every direction, affecting everyone and everything, for the duration of time. Let me provide an example:

One day a man was standing on the shore of a lake, skipping rocks. After a few successful throws, resulting in multiple skips, he noticed a teenager floating by in a kayak. The teenager didn't seem to notice the man but, instead, appeared to be leaning over and staring at something in the water.

The man was feeling playful, so he picked up a large rock and heaved it close to the side of the kayak, being careful to not actually hit the young lady, only startle her. It did startle her! So much so that she tipped over and fell into the lake. Suddenly the man felt bad for what he had done, so he dove into the lake, swam out to the her, righted the kayak, and helped her climb back in. Then the man apologized to her. She replied, "that's okay." And they parted ways.

The day before, that same girl had been kayaking with her dad. It was her first time to navigate a kayak on her own. At one point the dad rowed his kayak up beside hers and began to teasingly rock it. She immediately dropped her paddle and, in a state of panic, clutched both sides of the kayak. Her father laughed at her reaction and told her that she needed to trust that he wouldn't tip her over. Hearing this, she began to relax just as he resumed his tipping. Again, out of panic, she leaned in the opposite direction of his tipping, just as he let go, and she tumbled out of the kayak into the chilly depths of the lake. Terrified as she reemerged, gasping for air, she heard her father laughing hysterically. She had never felt so betrayed, especially by someone she was supposed to trust more than anyone. She wondered if she could ever trust a man again, much less trust a kayak. That night she lay awake, thinking to herself that her first step toward healing would be to take that kayak out again the next day.

That next day, as she pushed away from the shore, she once again felt the terror as the kayak initially rocked from her entry. But as she settled in, she began to relax a little and even began to enjoy the calm and beauty of the lake. After a while she stopped paddling for a moment to simply drift and take in her recovering courage. As she stared down into the water, she thought to herself, *Maybe I can trust my dad again. Surely men aren't all mean.* That's when she heard the splash.

Years later, she was married and had a child of her own. Her marriage was strained. Her husband felt like he always had to prove himself trustworthy to her. He couldn't understand why. It hurt. He felt unaccepted. What now made things worse was that she seemed to be passing her mistrust of him on to their child. The last straw for him came one day when they were at a hotel swimming pool with their child. His wife was reading a book as she lounged by the pool. He was in the shallow end with his five-year-old daughter sitting on the steps. He began to think to himself that it was about time he taught his daughter how to swim. But first, he thought, he would have to build her confidence in him.

"Let's see if you can jump off the side into the water, like *that* little boy is doing with his dad," he said to his daughter, as he pointed toward the dad and son a few feet away. "Don't worry. I'll catch you before your head goes under!"

"Okay daddy! Promise you'll catch me?" The little girl said as she climbed up the steps.

"Of course!" He replied. "You can trust me. I'm your daddy!"

Just then, the dad heard a frantic scream. He looked up to see his wife run up, scoop the little girl into her arms, and give him the coldest look he had ever seen on her face.

One year later, they were divorced.

As the little girl grew, her mother would look for opportunities to point out that men were not to be trusted. She taught her well, and years later, her little girl was now in a marriage that was strained because *she* didn't trust men.

Everything we do, good or bad, has consequences that not only last a lifetime, they affect everyone around us. And their children. And their grandchildren. And their grandchildren's children. We will never know all the ways our actions will affect the generations to come. This is another reason that forgiveness, between humans, is a process. There will be consequences, discovered along the way, that will need to be dealt with. For that young lady in the kayak to eventually heal, she will need to step into the process of forgiveness. For that man who threw the rock into the lake, simply apologizing does not make right the wrong he has done.

In the past, I have taught the process of forgiveness from two perspectives: the role of the offender and the role of the forgiver. Although there are some helpful tools that are specific to only one role or the other, what is really at the core, of both roles, is the need for contrition. If both sides are being contrite, there is no need to explain the tools. They will be picked up and used naturally. So, I am going to simply focus on the contrition.

Contrition is a word that is not even used by most people, much less understood. I'm not sure I even understand what all it entails, but here is what I've come up with so far:

Asking for forgiveness
Seeking to understand the full extent of the damage done
Conveying that understanding to those involved
Attempting to repair the damage
Taking a better path

Most of what I think contrition is about comes from Psalm 51, in the Old Testament. In this passage, David, the most famous King of Israel, says:

You do not delight in sacrifice, or I would bring it; you do not take pleasure in burnt offerings. My sacrifice, O God, is a broken spirit; a broken and contrite heart you, God, will not despise.

A loose translation: God isn't very interested in the things we do to right our wrongs. We will never be able to right them all in the first place. What God wants is for us to understand how devastating our wrong is and to take personal responsibility for that devastation. The things we do in attempt to right our wrongs are important! But, not to please God. Rather, those sacrifices help us to acknowledge the hurts we have caused. They should be an outward symbol of an inward conviction, which is the most important piece. Inward conviction is so profoundly important because without it, we are likely to repeat the action. If the man who threw the stone in the lake does not acknowledge that his action did more than startle the young lady in the kayak, what's to keep him from doing it again? Wasn't startling her the reason for doing so in the first place?

So first, if I am contrite, I start with asking for forgiveness. By definition, forgiveness is not deserved. If I expect my spouse to immediately respond with, "I forgive you," after I've asked for forgiveness, then I am not being contrite. Instead, I ask for forgiveness and, as I'm doing so, release it to her. She may pause for a moment before saying "I forgive you." Or, it may take a few days. She may never say it. But I must remember that she's not obligated to do so. I don't deserve her forgiveness. If I am remaining contrite, I leave that for her to decide. I don't stand there waiting for her response. By the way, the more she sees that I'm not requiring a positive response from her, the easier it will be for her to grant me that response. It's a process.

Second, if I am contrite, I am seeking to understand the full extent of the damage done. But I will never see all the damage that has been done, and there will still be consequences long after I'm gone. So, I will never fully accomplish this task. It's a process.

Third, if I am contrite, I am seeking to convey that understanding to those involved. Suppose I stole a hundred dollars from my neighbor. Three days later my feelings of conviction are too much, so I go to him, ask for his forgiveness, and pay him back. But a week later I learn that when he discovered the money was missing, he wrongfully accused his son of stealing it. Doing so deeply affected their relationship. Don't I have the responsibility to explain to his son that it was my fault and seek his forgiveness as well, even though his father already forgave me? Of course I do! Forgiveness is a process.

Fourth, if I am contrite, I am seeking to repair the damage I've done as I discover that damage along the way. Let's suppose I stole Timmy's lunch money one day when we were in second grade. One day, when I'm forty years old, something occurs that reminds me of that deed. But Timmy might be dead for all I know. Even if he's still alive, I don't know Timmy's last name. Am I supposed to quit my job and leave my family to go on a quest to find Timmy and pay him back? Of course not! But, if I have a contrite heart, then when I see a child crying because a bully has just taken her lunch money, I can hand her a few dollars and show her I understand what it's like to be in her shoes.

Fifth, if I am contrite, I am on a different path than the one I was on when I committed the offense. Speaking of-fences (I hope you appreciate my poetic wordplay), suppose I was throwing rocks at my fence which stands between my neighbor and myself, just for pitching practice. One of those rocks slips and hits my neighbor's window, leaving it shattered. So, I apologize, and have it repaired. The next day I go right back to that rock pile and resume my pitching practice, throwing rocks toward that same spot on the fence. Why would it bother me that my neighbor is standing out in his yard, staring at me with crossed arms? Of course, he believes that it is likely to happen again. And the reason he has a scowl on his face is because I'm apparently not contrite.

Forgiveness is a process because for the offender, it requires contrition. Contrition is not an action. Contrition is a heart condition that calls us to action. It is a way of being, not an action that happens in a moment.

At face value, then, contrition would be a lifelong process that becomes an ever-increasing burden. The more we wrong people, the more we have to seek to understand the damage done. The more damage we find, the more people we have to convey that understanding to those we've wronged. The more damage we discover, the more repairing we have to do. Soon, there would be no time to do anything else. Even if we were to spend all our time doing this, it would just keep piling up, becoming a bigger and bigger burden that is impossible to bear. It would crush your spirit, that is, if forgiveness is something that happens in a moment in time and if it's more about something you do than a way of being.

But, if a contrite heart is, instead, something that we are striving more and more toward, and we believe in a thing I will call *unconditional universal grace*, then that load is constantly being lifted. Instead of walking through life with an ever-increasing load of guilt and shame, with unconditional universal grace, we understand ourselves to be forgiven before we even commit a hurtful deed. With unconditional universal grace, we are forgiven even if we never ask for it. This is the grace that God extends to all of us, whether we receive it or not. It is offered whether or not we acknowledge we need it. It is granted to us, whether or not we acknowledge it. The reason we are to ask for forgiveness from God is *not* so that God will grant it, that's already been done. The reason we are to ask is that, in asking, we acknowledge that we need it. If we don't even acknowledge that we need it, why would we receive it? God does not *require* our asking in order that God grant us forgiveness. God invites us to ask so that we will receive it and, in receiving, walk through life without the unbearable burden of the destruction our deeds have brought to ourselves and others. The more we walk through life in this *unconditional universal grace*, the lighter our step is, the higher we hold our head, the more joyful we are, and the quicker we are to forgive, even when we aren't asked for it. We don't withhold forgiveness from our spouses, waiting for them to ask or be sincerely contrite. We are just passing on the grace that is constantly flowing to ourselves.

But you may tell yourself that you don't need something like this. You don't need forgiveness to be a process or contrition to be your way of life, because you don't carry grudges. Furthermore, when you've done wrong, you forgive yourself immediately and move on with no regrets, even when others don't forgive you. You don't have to carry a weight around, and you don't need some sort of cosmic grace to make you feel better about yourself.

If that's the case, I have some questions that need explaining:

How do you forgive someone who has wrongfully fired you from a job? If you haven't fully forgiven them, why not?

How do you forgive someone who has cheated on you but has not asked for your forgiveness? If you haven't fully forgiven them, how do you justify that you deserve forgiveness for the hurts you have caused others?

How do you forgive someone who has sexually molested you but hasn't acknowledged it?

If you haven't fully forgiven him or her, what is your standard for what is unforgiveable and what is not?

In other words, if you haven't fully forgiven everyone who has ever wronged you, how can you fully forgive yourself?

You can't.

And, as much as you try to trick your mind into thinking you are forgiven, you won't be able to. Your misdeeds will keep piling up on you, eventually becoming a burden that is too heavy to carry. You might experience it by becoming more and more depressed or more and more anxious. You might experience it by becoming more and more bitter and angry. What is almost sure to happen is that you will not be able to maintain life-long relationships that continue to grow and thrive. Instead, you will find yourself becoming more and more resentful toward anyone you invest your life into. Because, ultimately, there will be times when they hurt you as well.

The process of forgiveness, lifelong contrition, is a life of ever-increasing freedom!

WHAT IT'S ALL ABOUT

What It's All About

I've talked a lot about acceptance in this book. It is at the core of what it means to love. My personal opinion is that love is at the core of what makes everything work well for, and among, human beings. The more accepting (loving) we our of our mate, the better our marriage is and the more likely we are to have a vibrant relationship that lasts a lifetime. The more accepting we are of our children, the more they turn to us, instead of seeking acceptance through gangs or misguided peers or social media. The more accepting we are of our neighbors, the more they watch out for us and support us, instead of complaining about our dog that tends to bark at harmless things at two o'clock in the morning. The more accepting we are of our coworkers and customers, the easier our jobs are and the more successful we are. The more accepting we are of the person who rails against our beliefs and ideas on Facebook, the less we become divided into ever-increasing polarization that tears our culture apart. The more accepting we are of people from other parts of the world, especially the ones who collectively want to harm us, the less they want to harm us and make war with us.

We are in a relationship with everyone on this planet. That doesn't mean that we know everyone or will even meet everyone, of course. But my actions effect everyone who comes in contact with me, whether it be in a real-life conversation with the cashier at the grocery store or someone who reads my Instagram post halfway around the world, whom I've never met. This international relationship dynamic has always been the case. However, with the fast-growing pace of technology, we are becoming more and more connected every year. Now, more than ever, our need to step up our acceptance game is crucial for our own well-being and those we care about. Our children's future depends on our acceptance becoming more at the core of how we interact with people, starting with their other parent and extending to everyone we encounter, whether it be personally or digitally.

To accept someone does not always mean to accept their behavior. In fact, accepting someone sometimes means that you need to confront them in order to effectively deal with any issues which may be adversely affecting the relationship. However, whether it is your spouse or the person in the next lane with a bumper sticker that states they are against what you believe in, they will not receive your confrontation with open ears unless they first believe that you accept them as a human being. And no one is going to believe that you accept them if they believe you think you are somehow better than them.

There is a passage in the Bible, specifically the New Testament, that gives us the parable of the "Good Samaritan." Many, who don't even attempt to follow the Bible, still know the basic story because it conveys a belief that is somewhat universal and applies to many faiths and philosophies for good living—to help people in need, especially when others won't. But there is so much else going on in this passage that reveals so much more when we look at it a little closer and see it more in the context in which it was written. So, let's look at some of the historical and cultural context first.

At the time, somewhere around 30 AD, the part of the world that is now known as Palestine and Israel was under Roman rule. The majority of people living there, like today, were Jewish and were hoping for and waiting on a Messiah. Most of them believed that this Messiah would be one of their own and a political and military type leader who would raise up an army to run the Romans out and take over as head of the government, restoring their own kingdom. But as Jesus began to teach, much of what he said seemed to go against what they wanted to hear. Furthermore, he wasn't saying anything that sounded like he was inspiring anyone to take up arms and revolt against the Romans, quite the contrary. His message seemed to be more about taking care of the helpless, feeding the poor, and befriending the outcast, instead of exploiting them, as many of the upper-class Jews were doing.

So, a lot of these upper-class Jews, known as Pharisees and Sadducees, began to confront Jesus in front of his followers, who believed he was the Messiah. All throughout the four accounts of Jesus (Matthew, Mark, Luke, John), we are shown instances of this. One of those accounts, in the book of Matthew, has the Pharisees get together and interrupt him while he is teaching his followers. One of them asks Jesus which commandment is the greatest. He already knows the answer, but he's hoping Jesus doesn't so that it would be obvious to everyone that he can't be the Messiah. In fact, any good and faithful Jew would know the answer to this guy's question. It's basically the Scripture known as the *Shema*. If you don't know the Shema, you're not even a Jew. In fact, everyone had it posted on their front door. Even today, practicing Jews have it on their front door, inside a little box called a *mezuzah*. You quoted it out loud when you got up in the morning and before you went to sleep. You told it to your children every day, twice a day. Here's what Jesus answered…

"Love the Lord your God with all your heart and with all your soul and with all your mind. This is the first and greatest commandment." Then he continued with another passage they would all know and believe to be very important. "And the second is like it: Love your neighbor as yourself."

It didn't work. Jesus knew the answer. Again, they failed to make him look bad. But Jesus wasn't finished. He went on…

"All the Law and the prophets hang on these two commandments."

What he is saying here is that all of Scripture is about these two commandments.

Further on, in Luke 10, we see it again. Another one of them comes up to Jesus, and, trying to test him to make him look bad in front of the others, he asks a similar question, "What do I have to do to have the life that lasts?"

Jesus turns it back on him, instead of answering it. "What is written in the Law?" Jesus replies. "How do you read it?"

He answered, "Love the Lord your God with all your heart and with all your soul and with all your strength and with all your mind. And, love your neighbor as yourself."

"You have answered correctly," Jesus replied. "Do this and you will have life."

Again, they didn't trap Jesus. Strike two. So, the guy tries again. "So, who is my neighbor?"

Jesus' reply was the parable of the Good Samaritan, which I will paraphrase and add some context to it as well.

There's this guy on the road from Jerusalem to Jericho…[1]

Jesus continues…

So as this guy is walking along, some robbers jumped him; beat him unconscious; stole his iPhone, his wallet, and his clothes; and left him there for dead. Then along comes a priest…

This is important information! He's basically saying, "One of your group comes along… one of you Pharisees or Sadducees who are always trying to make me look bad. That priest comes along and does nothing for the guy. He moves around him and then goes on his merry way."

Then a Levite comes along and does the same thing… he doesn't stop to help.

---

[1] Today, there are actually two roads going from Jerusalem to Jericho, the more recent high road and the ancient low road through the canyon. The low road is the one he is speaking of. About twenty years ago, Joanna and I were on a tour bus on the high road. At one point we pulled over and got a look at the lower road. The tour guide told us all that, to this day, there's a good chance you'll get robbed if you walk down the low road alone.

A priest *is* a Levite! He's essentially saying that another one of you sees this man dying, and it doesn't even bother him enough to stop and see if he can help in any way. Can you imagine? Nobody else is around to help him and he's obviously badly wounded! The story continues…

Finally, a Samaritan comes along, stops, gives him first aid, puts him in his car, drives him to town to the hospital, takes him in, and pays his medical bills until he's all better.

Now is when it's really getting good. The moment he said the word "Samaritan," their attention would have been grabbed by both hands and the hair would have stood up on the back of their necks. Samaritans were considered, by Jews at that time, as the scum of the earth. They were worse than pagans because they mixed the Jewish religion with other religions. Historians, who lived at the time of Jesus, tell us that when a Jew saw a Samaritan walking down the street toward him, the Jew would cross the street and walk on the other side, so as not to be within touching distance, not to mention conversation distance. Jesus knows what he's doing here. He knows his peripheral audience will be upset. That's the reason for his extreme example! So, he then asks the man who tried to set him up…

Which of these three do you think was a neighbor to the man who fell into the hands of the robbers?

To which the other man replied, "The one who had mercy on him." Jesus drops the proverbial mic… "Go and do likewise."

That question—who is my neighbor—is key here. By this time, these Pharisees and Sadducees had been watching Jesus for quite some time. They had confronted him for hanging out with "sinners" instead of "good churchgoing, Scripture-following folks." In their culture, someone who didn't avoid all of the taboos they avoided, who didn't worship with them in their synagogue, and who didn't dress like them and think like them, those people were not allowed to live in their community—they weren't their *neighbors*! Jesus totally flips this one on them. You've got it wrong! Your neighbor is whoever is in your path. Whoever! It doesn't take real love to hang out and care for people who are just like you… that's just self-preservation. You're not loving me unless you are treating *all* my children (humans) like you would treat yourself! Furthermore, you're not loving God if you don't love *all* his children!

When Jesus says that all the law and the prophets hang on these two commands, love God with all you got and love your neighbor as yourself, he's saying that all the other commands in Scripture fall under these two commands. They "hang" below them. Yet you people keep trying to turn things upside down. You go to great pains to make sure you are keeping all the rules, but you are ignoring the game that the rules are all about—love!

During that two-week tour Joanna and I took, we spent a few nights in the town of Nazareth, Jesus' home town. We got there late one Friday afternoon, and as the bus pulled up to the hotel, the tour guide announced that we were running a little late. So, he told us to hurry, get checked in, get our luggage up to our room, and be back down stairs in twenty minutes for dinner. As I recall, our room was on the eighth floor. After we got checked in and were given our key, the two of us went down the hall and stepped into the elevator. When we turned around, we noticed that some mischievous kid had pushed all the buttons. It was like in the movie *Elf* where Will Ferrell, in his childlike enthusiasm, lit up all the buttons on the Empire State Building elevator.

Thank goodness we didn't have to go up one hundred floors, but it was, nonetheless, somewhat annoying to have to stop on every floor, wait for the doors to open and see nobody there waiting, and then pause for the doors to close again and move on to the next floor, only to experience the same thing again, floor after floor!

Finally, we reached the eighth floor, put our bags in our room, freshened up a bit, and then headed back down the hall to the elevator. We pushed the "down arrow" button and waited longer than I have ever waited for an elevator. When it finally arrived, we stepped in and guess what… the same kid had done it again! All the buttons were lit up and we had to stop on every floor on the way down. And no one was there waiting to get on.

When we finally made it down to the restaurant, we apologized to the group for being late and explained ourselves: "You wouldn't believe it! On both the way up to our room, and the way down, some little kid has pushed all the buttons, so it took us at least eight times as long to get here!"

"That happened to us all," one person in the group responded. "It's the Sabbath. The elevators are programmed to stop on every floor on the Sabbath so that no one does the work of pushing buttons. Remember, you're not supposed to work on the Sabbath. You're supposed to rest!"

What in the wide, wide world of sports? I could have gotten fifteen more minutes of rest if I could have taken the two seconds to push that button! My heart just had to work four times as hard to deal with the frustration and anxiety! What sort of religious crap is this? Wouldn't it be a lot more loving to let me push my own button than to make me wait for the elevator to stop on every floor? If the manager of that hotel was truly trying to follow the Shema, first and foremost, wouldn't he have let me push the buttons?

Yet, I often find myself being that hotel manager to my wife, as well as those around me. I put my so-called *principle*s above my relationships. It comes in many forms:

- Arguing my political perspective instead of listening to theirs in order to understand
- Demanding my way because it is the "right" way
- Posting polarizing and inflammatory statements on social media so I don't have to have real, loving conversations with people who don't think like me
- Wearing T-shirts that make strong religious statements so that people who don't believe like me won't bother me or so I can lure them into an argument
- Telling someone "I'll pray *for* you" instead of being *with* them when they need a friend, because it's too uncomfortable for me or because I'd rather spend my time doing "holy" stuff

These are just other forms of what Jesus is addressing here. Doing them makes us feel righteous because we fool ourselves into thinking we are being better than them or that we are standing up for our faith. Well, God doesn't need us to stand up for God. God doesn't call us to stand up for God. God calls us to love.

And here is one of the biggest reasons I'm so passionate about marriage: If I can't love my spouse, then I can't really love anyone. If my love for my spouse is based on the way he or she thinks or behaves, then that becomes my standard for love itself. If I spend a significant part of my life with anyone, I am going to encounter things I don't agree with them on. They will behave in ways I think are wrong. They are going to hurt me. Eventually, I will stop loving them as well, because my love is based on their actions and/or ideas. That's not love. That's coercion—to try to change them into something I want.

I believe it is really important to make something clear about everything I've written so far... I fail, miserably, every day! But what I strive to do, every day, is thank God that Joanna doesn't expect me to be the ideal husband... there's no such thing. Additionally, there's no such thing as the ideal wife. We are all humans. We all have issues. We all do hurtful things. We all have bad habits. But, if you are thinking about getting your significant other to read this book, let me give you some helpful advice: burn it![2]

Because, if you are putting your hopes in the idea that this book will help that person make you feel more loved, you've missed the entire point. That is not acceptance. That is not love. Instead, why don't you let them see you living out this book, more and more every day? Then, one day, if they ask you what has changed you so much, why you seem to love them so much better, you can point to this book as something that nudged you in that direction. But that day may never even need to come. If you are living out true acceptance, you won't feel like you need the other to change in order to be a whole, healthy, joyful person.

---

[2] But, don't let that stop you from buying a dozen copies to give to friends who know you accept them!

So, I will end with this:

The core of what drives us is the desire to be accepted.

No one is acceptable on the basis of their behavior.

Choosing to love is choosing to accept, regardless of behavior.

This is the love that God extends to you, whether you accept it or not.

This is the love that God intends for you to pass on to all his children

… especially your spouse.

Epilogue

Remember a few chapters back when I wrote about power struggles and choosing restaurants? Often, when I present that in a seminar or speaking engagement, I will get a question like this:

"Sure, I can see this working for things like choosing a restaurant. But, what about the things that really matter to you, matters that have to do with your moral convictions and values. You know, things that you don't believe you should compromise on?"

So, let me throw in one more story that blew my mind and changed my heart.

I was conducting a seminar in the Midwest and had just given this restaurant example, of sharing power, when one of the husbands in attendance raised his hand and asked that same question: "Sure, I can see this working for things like choosing a restaurant. But, what about the things that really matter to you, matters that have to do with your moral convictions and values. You know, things that you don't believe you should compromise on?"

I answered by saying that sharing power has, so far, worked with every issue that Joanna and I had encountered, since we began to apply it.

"I just don't see how it can work in our situation," he replied. "You see, I'm a devout Muslim and my wife is a devout Christian. We have three boys, ages three, five, and seven. I believe that the boys should attend our mosque with me. My wife believes they should attend church with her.

How do we take our penny off the table when we each truly believe that it is the only acceptable one?"

I about pooped my pants.

But my back was against the proverbial wall in front of all these people who had paid good money to get help with their marriages. No doubt, they had in mind their own issues that they couldn't see as something they could compromise upon. So, I stalled for time… I presented a template that can be used when you run up against the really tough issues. It looks like this:

1. Identify the issue from both perspectives, giving equal time to both perspectives.
2. Brainstorm every possible solution you can think of (look for every penny you can find).
3. Together, choose the one that best satisfies both of your concerns.

I then started with step one. We did a coin toss to see which spouse would go first. The wife won the coin toss, so I told her she has two minutes to explain her concerns. She then proceeded to make a passionate, convicted speech about why the boys should attend church with her. After two minutes were up, the husband then gave a convicted, passionate speech about why the boys should attend the mosque with him. Then, I announced that since both spouses seem to only see the two options, or pennies, the entire group would help them see some of the proverbial pennies on the floor, as I wrote what they suggested on the board.

After about fifteen minutes, we had filled the entire board with ideas:

Alternate weeks
Let the boys decide
Attend a Universalist Church
Attend no church
Get a divorce (which wouldn't have solved the problem)
Have them attend school at one and worship at the other

Call a meeting of the Pastor and the Imam for their input
Go to the mosque on Saturdays and to church on Sundays

These were just some of the suggestions. After we filled the board, we voted for the top three. As I circled those three suggestions, I saw my way out of the situation.

"Well, there are three really good suggestions! Write them down and take them home. And, together, choose the one that works best for both of you."

One of the first questions I usually get, when I tell this story, is why they got married to each other in the first place. Now you have an answer to that question. It's called "limerence," when two people say, "We're in love! It doesn't matter because this is true love!"

Yes, when they met, they were already involved in their separate faiths. In fact, up until this time, he had never stepped foot on the grounds of her church. And, she had never stepped foot on the grounds of his mosque.[3] Over time, he had become firmly entrenched in the *overt power* position, concerning this issue. And, she had settled into the *covert power* position. He would defiantly declare that he was the head of the household and take them to the mosque on the Saturdays he was in town. But his job required him being out of town on many weekends. On those particular weekends, she would take the boys to church and whisper not to tell their father. Of course, he would find out now and then, and the issue became a bigger and bigger wedge between them, to the point that the oldest, only seven years old, had recently announced that as soon as he was old enough, he was leaving home and wasn't going to have anything to do with either of their faiths. All he could see about their faiths was the way they used them to hurt each other.

A week later, I received an email from that couple. They explained what happened a few days after they got home.

---

[3] Occasionally, when I tell this story, someone will point out to me that, in traditional Islam, women are not allowed in the mosque. While that is true, most mosques have adjacent facilities for women and children to worship and learn The Koran.

Together, they sat the boys down, and the mother began by telling them that she did not condone or support her husband's faith. However, because he is her husband, she is going to support him as a person and, in turn, support the family by attending the mosque with them on Saturdays.

Then, the father announced that he did not condone or support his wife's faith. However, because she is his wife, he is going to support her as a person and, in turn, support the family by attending the church with her on Sundays.

About six months later, we received a card from them, with a picture of the whole family smiling around the dinner table. They said that their marriage was now stronger than it had ever been. "And, oh, by the way," the husband wrote on the back, "last week I was baptized."

I doubt that would have happened had they continued to put their principles above their relationships. When they chose to truly accept each other, when they realized they didn't have to accept the others' beliefs and practices to accept the person, they created a space for God to move in and help them live out the greatest commandment, the one that all the other commandments are about: love God and love your neighbor—**the acceptance**.

SOURCES

Axinn, William G. and Thornton, Arland (1992). The relationship between cohabitation and divorce: Selectivity or causal influence? *Demography, 29*, 357–374.

Brown, Susan L. and Booth, Alan (1996). Cohabitation versus marriage: A comparison of relationship quality. *Journal of Marriage and the Family, 58*, 668–678.

Bumpass, Larry L. and Sweet, James (1989). National estimates of cohabitation. *Demography, 26*, 615–626.

Chapman, Gary (2015). *The Five Love Languages: The Secret to Love that Lasts.* Chicago. Northfield Publishing

Cohan, C. L. and Kleinbaum, S. (2002). Toward a greater understanding of the Cohabitation effect: Premarital cohabitation and marital communication. *Journal of Marriage and Family, 64*, 180–192.

DeMaris, A. and Leslie, G. R. (1984). Cohabitation with future spouse: Its influence upon marital satisfaction and communication. *Journal of Marriage and Family, 46*, 77–84.

Forste, R. and Tanfer, K. (1996). Sexual exclusivity among dating, cohabiting, and married women. *Journal of Marriage and the Family, 58*, 594–600.

Feldhahn, Shaunti (2014). *The Good News About Marriage: Debunking Discouraging Myths About Marriage and Divorce.* Colorado Springs, Colorado. Multnomah books

Harley, Willard R., Jr. (2011) *His Needs Her Needs: Building an Affair-Proof Marriage*. Grand Rapids, Michigan. Revell

Kahneman, Daniel & Deaton, Angus (2010). High Income Improves Evaluation of Life But Not Emotional Well Being. *Proceedings of the National Academy of Sciences of the United States of America, 107(38):16489–93*

Kamp Dush, C. M.; Cohan, C. L.; & Amato, P. R. (2003). The relationship between cohabitation and marital quality and stability: Change across cohorts? *Journal of Marriage and Family, 65*, 539–549.

Kline, G. H.; Stanley, S. M.; Markman, H. J.; Olmos-Gallo, P. A.; St. Peters, M.; Whitton, S. W.; Prado, L. (2004). Timing is everything: Pre-engagement cohabitation and increased risk for poor marital outcomes. *Journal of Family Psychology, 18*, 311–318.

Laumann, Edward O.; Gagnon, John H.; Michael, Robert T.; Michaels, Stuart (1994). *The Social Organization of Sexuality: Sexual Practices in the United States*. Chicago: University of Chicago Press.

Maslow, A. H. (1943). A Theory of Human Motivation. *Psychological Review*. 30, 370–396

McManus, Mike and McManus, Harriet (2008). *Living Together: Myths, Risks & Answers*. New York: Howard Books.

Rhoades, G. K.; Stanley, S. M.; & Markman, H. J. (2009). The pre-engagement cohabitation effect: A replication and extension of previous findings. *Journal of Family Psychology, 30*, 233–258.

Rhoades, G. K.; Stanley, S. M.; & Markman, H. J. (2009). Couples' reasons for cohabitation: Associations with individual well-being and relationship quality. *Journal of Family Issues, 30*, 233–258.

Short, Doug (2016). Happiness Revisited: A Household Income of $75K?. Advisor Perspectives, October 21, 2016

Smith, T.W. (2006). American Sexual Behavior: Trends, Socio-Demographic Differences, and Risk Behavior. *GSS Topical Report No. 25*. Chicago.

Stanley, S. M.; Rhoades, G. K.; Amato, P. R.; Markman, H. J.; & Johnson,

C. A. (2010). The timing of cohabitation and engagement: Impact on first and second marriages. *Journal of Marriage and Family, 72*, 906–918.

Stanley, S. M.; Rhoades, G. K.; & Markman, H. J. (2006). Sliding vs. Deciding: Inertia and the premarital cohabitation effect. *Family Relations, 55*, 499–509.

Stanley, S.M.; Whitton, S. W.; & Markman, H. J. (2004). Maybe I do: Interpersonal commitment and premarital or nonmarital cohabitation. *Journal of Family Issues, 25*, 496–519.

Stanley, S. (1998). *The heart of commitment: Compelling research that reveals the secrets of a lifelong, intimate marriage.* Nashville: Thomas Nelson.

Stets, J. E. and Strous, M. A. (1989). The marriage license as a hitting license: A comparison of assaults in dating, cohabiting, and married couples *Journal of Family Violence, 4*(2), 161–180.

Tennov, Dorothy (1999). *Love and Limerence: The Experience of Being in Love.* Lanham, Maryland. Scarborough House

Thomson, Elizabeth and Colella, Ugo (1992). Cohabitation and marital stability: Quality or commitment? *Journal of Marriage and the Family, 54*, 259–267.

Thornton, Arland (1988).Cohabitation and marriage in the 1980s. *Demography, 25*, 497–508.

Waite, Linda J. and Joyner, Kara (1996). Men's and women's general happiness and sexual satisfaction in marriage, cohabitation, and single living. Paper presented to the *Population Research Center's Demography Workshop.*

Waite, Linda J.; Browning, Don; Doherty, W. J.; Gallagher, Maggie; Luo, Ye; & Stanley, Scott M. (2002). Does Divorce Make People Happy?: Findings from a Study of Unhappy Marriages, Press Release

Does Divorce Make People Happy?

Findings from a Study of Unhappy Marriages

By Linda J. Waite, Don Browning, William J. Doherty, Maggie Gallagher, Ye Luo, and Scott M. Stanley

Press Release
Embargoed Until July 11, 2002, 10:00 AM EST
Contact: Mary Schwarz, T. (212) 246-3942
Major New Study:

Call it the "divorce assumption." Most people assume that a person stuck in a bad marriage has two choices: stay married and miserable or get a divorce and become happier.[1] But now come the findings from the first scholarly study ever to test that assumption, and these findings challenge conventional wisdom. Conducted by a team of leading family scholars headed by University of Chicago sociologist Linda Waite, the study found no evidence that unhappily married adults who divorced were typically any happier than unhappily married people who stayed married.

Even more dramatically, the researchers also found that two-thirds of unhappily married spouses who stayed married reported that their marriages were happy five years later. In addition, the most unhappy marriages reported the most dramatic turnarounds: among those who rated their marriages as very unhappy, almost eight out of ten who avoided divorce were happily married five years later.[2]

The research team used data collected by the National Survey of Families and Households, a nationally representative survey that extensively measures personal and marital happiness. Out of 5,232 married adults interviewed in the late eighties, 645 reported being unhappily married. Five years later, these same adults were interviewed again. Some had divorced or separated and some had stayed married.

The study found that on average unhappily married adults who divorced were no happier than unhappily married adults who stayed married when rated on any of twelve separate measures of psychological well-being. Divorce did not typically reduce symptoms of depression, raise self-esteem, or increase a sense of mastery. This was true even after controlling for race, age, gender, and income. Even unhappy spouses who had divorced and remarried were no happier on average than those who stayed married. "Staying married is not just for the children's sake. Some divorce is necessary, but results like these suggest the benefits of divorce have been oversold," says Linda J. Waite.

Why doesn't divorce typically make adults happier? The authors of the study suggest that while eliminating some stresses and sources of potential harm, divorce may create others as well. The decision to divorce sets in motion a large number of processes and events over which an individual has little control that are likely to deeply affect his or her emotional well-being. These include the response of one's spouse to divorce; the reactions of children; potential disappointments and aggravation in custody, child support, and visitation orders; new financial or health stresses for one or both parents; and new relationships or marriages. The team of family experts that conducted the study included Linda J. Waite; Lucy Flower, professor of sociology at The University of Chicago and coauthor of *The Case for Marriage*; Don Browning, professor emeritus of the University of Chicago Divinity School; William J. Doherty, professor of family social science and director of the Marriage and Family Therapy program at the University of Minnesota; Maggie Gallagher, affiliate scholar at the Institute for American Values and coauthor of *The Case for Marriage*; Ye Luo, a research associate at the Sloan Center on Parents, Children and Work at The University of Chicago; and Scott Stanley, codirector of the Center for Marital and Family Studies at the University of Denver.

Marital Turnarounds: How Do Unhappy Marriages Get Happier?

To follow up on the dramatic findings that two-thirds of unhappy marriages had become happy five years later, the researchers also conducted focus group interviews with fifty-five formerly unhappy husbands and wives who had turned their marriages around. They found that many currently happily married spouses have had extended periods of marital unhappiness, often for quite serious reasons, including alcoholism, infidelity, verbal abuse, emotional neglect, depression, illness, and work reversals.

Why did these marriages survive where other marriages did not? Spouses' stories of how their marriages got happier fell into three broad headings: the marital endurance ethic, the marital work ethic, and the personal happiness ethic.

In the marital endurance ethic, the most common story couples reported to researchers is that marriages got happier not because partners resolved problems, but because they stubbornly outlasted them. With the passage of time, these spouses said many sources of conflict and distress eased: financial problems, job reversals, depression, child problems, and even infidelity. In the marital work ethic, spouses told stories of actively working to solve problems, change behavior, or improve communication. When the problem was solved, the marriage got happier. Strategies for improving marriages mentioned by spouses ranged from arranging dates or other ways to more time together, to enlisting the help and advice of relatives or in-laws, to consulting clergy or secular counselors, to threatening divorce and consulting divorce attorneys. Finally, in the personal happiness epic, marriage problems did not seem to change that much. Instead married people in these accounts told stories of finding alternative ways to improve their own happiness and build a good and happy life despite a mediocre marriage.

The Powerful Effects of Commitment

Spouses interviewed in the focus groups whose marriages had turned around generally had a low opinion of the benefits of divorce, as well as friends and family members who supported the importance of staying married. Because of their intense commitment to their marriages, these couples invested great effort in enduring or overcoming problems in their relationships, they minimized the importance of difficulties they couldn't resolve, and they actively worked to belittle the attractiveness of alternatives.

The study's findings are consistent with other research demonstrating the powerful effects of marital commitment on marital happiness. A strong commitment to marriage as an institution and a powerful reluctance to divorce do not merely keep unhappily married people locked in misery together. They also help couples form happier bonds. To avoid divorce, many assume, marriages must become happier. But it is at least equally true that in order to get happier, unhappy couples or spouses must first avoid divorce. "In most cases, a strong commitment to staying married not only helps couples avoid divorce, it helps more couples achieve a happier marriage," notes research team member Scott Stanley.

Would most unhappy spouses who divorced have ended up happily married if they had stuck with their marriages?

The researchers who conducted the study cannot say for sure whether unhappy spouses who divorced would have become happy had they stayed with their marriages. In most respects, unhappy spouses who divorced and unhappy spouses who stayed married looked more similar than different (before the divorce) in terms of their psychological adjustment and family background. While unhappy spouses who divorced were on average younger, had lower household incomes, and were more likely to be employed or to have children in the home, these differences were typically not large.

Were the marriages that ended in divorce much worse than those that did not? There is some evidence for this point of view. Unhappy spouses who divorced reported more conflict and were about twice as likely to report violence in their marriage than unhappy spouses who stayed married. However, marital violence occurred in only a minority of unhappy marriages: twenty-one percent of unhappy spouses who divorced reported husband-to-wife violence, compared to nine percent of unhappy spouses who stayed married.

On the other hand, if only the worst marriages ended up in divorce, one would expect divorce to be associated with important psychological benefits. Instead, researchers found that unhappily married adults who divorced were no more likely to report emotional and psychological improvements than those who stayed married. In addition, the most unhappy marriages reported the most dramatic turnarounds: among those who rated their marriages as very unhappy, almost eight out of ten who avoided divorce were happily married five years later.

More research is needed to establish under what circumstances divorce improves or lessens adult well-being, as well as what kinds of unhappy marriages are most or least likely to improve if divorce is avoided.

Other Findings

Other findings of the study based on the National Survey Data are the following:

The vast majority of divorces (seventy-four percent) took place to adults who had been happily married when first studied five years earlier. In this group, divorce was associated with dramatic declines in happiness and psychological well-being compared to those who stayed married. Unhappy marriages are less common than unhappy spouses; three out of four unhappily married adults are married to someone who is happy with the marriage. Staying married did not typically trap unhappy spouses in violent relationships. Eighty-six percent of unhappily married adults reported no violence in their relationship (including seventy-seven percent of unhappy spouses who later divorced or separated). Ninety-three percent of unhappy spouses who avoided divorce reported no violence in their marriage five years later.

Thanks to...

Joanna, if I had to do it all over again, you'd still be my first choice. Everyday I hope you feel the same.

Dad, you taught me that loving all people is the core of life.

Mom, you are an amazing woman! The way you and dad continue to make your lives be about loving everyone, especially the ones who need it most, continues to be my compass.

Abby, what a dream it is to get to go to the "office" every day with my oldest daughter.

Connor, my only son, the way you treat waiters and grocery store cashiers, shows that you get what life is about.

Ana, those 4th graders, who get to spend 5 days a week with you, don't know how blessed they are.

Carter & Jackson, I couldn't have asked for better sons-in-law.

Anderson Duke Jennings, the world became brighter April 3, 2019!

For making this book happen...

Randy Boggs for keeping me going. Christopher Anderson for the cover photo and being a great brother for 49 years. Steve Green, for showing me the landscape. Laura Minchew, for showing me the ropes. Max Lucado, for your inspiration, encouragement, and support. David Chatham, for your input and all the stuff you edited over the years for practically free. Darrell Smith, for helping me believe I could make it happen. Paul Soupiset, for the awesome cover and illustration. Carl Caton, you are a rare gem. Gabi Powell, the best writer I know, and actually liked the book. Brian Martindale, Bill Earle, Xandra, and the rest of the great people at Elm Hill.

My Family that loves like crazy...

Michele & Wes English, Travis & Kirsten English, Shaylea & Matthew McMillan, Shiloh, Tabin, Sawyer

Debbie & Randy Boggs, Andress & Alex Eichstadt, Caitlin & Josh Lee, Grey, Asher, Keyes, Ramsey, Ebby

Christopher Anderson, Marion Durand, Atlas, Pia

Bob Gomez (Popi) thanks for raising my wife so well. Nana, I miss you!

Russell & Gina Harrison, Hunter & Taylor Harrison, Marshall & Kennedi Harrison, Kennedy Harrison, Cannon

Dan & Tante Powell, Gabi Powell, Landon Powell

Mark & Ellen Abshier, Max & Denalyn Lucado, Steve & Cheryl Green, Preston & Julie Woolfolk, Lori Dawson, Andy & Missy Ivankovich, Chuck Cammack, Eliot & Julie Young, Tim Russo, Carlos & Nora Rodriguez, Dionna Sanchez, Anna Panter, all the folks at San Antonio Marriage Initiative, Dave Galbraith, Chad Warner, Bob Rauscher, Jonathan Daugherty, Dinah Shelly, Patricia Adams, David Karney, Sarah & John Dale, Tim & Suzie Dudich, Jon Mullican, Grady King, Hope Network, Cindy (Squeeky) Walker, John Isom, Cindy Downs, The Junction Boys, The Connections team, Oak Hills Church, The Tuesday night group: David Brigham, Randy Boggs, William Melendez (miss you)

Our Life Group of More than 20 years: John & Carol, David & Tristi, Steve & Mary, David & Josie. And, to all the many people who have supported Growing Love Network over the years... thanks for believing in what we do!

About the Author

J on R Anderson is the founder and president of Growing Love Network, a 501c3 non-profit organization dedicated to revolutionizing relationships for lifelong love. Jon earned his Master's degree in Marriage and Family Therapy in 1997 from Abilene Christian University. Since that time he has worked with thousands of couples and individuals through his counseling, workshops, and sem- 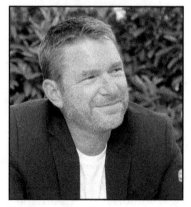 inars. Jon also has 18 years experience teaching college psychology and student development courses. He formerly served as the Coordinator of Counseling Services at San Antonio College, and as adjunct professor at Northwest Vista College. Jon is best know for leading more than 125 marriage intensive workshops, *Love Reboot*, and his podcast, *Relationship Rewire*, which gets more than 50,000 downloads per month. He is the author of *Growing Love* and *365 Days of Growing Love*.

Jon has been married to Joanna since 1985. They have 3 children, two sons-in-law, and 3 grand-dogs. In April of 2019, their wonderful first grandchild, *Anderson*, was born.

Our 3-day intensive workshop, *Love Reboot*, has helped thousands turn their failing marriages around.

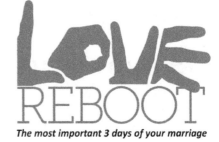

The most important 3 days of your marriage

RELATIONSHIP REWIRE

with **Jon R Anderson**

Our podcast, *Relationship Rewire*, has been downloaded over one million times. With numerous, well-known guests, Jon R Anderson talks about what we get wrong, and what we get right, when it comes to relationships and marriage in our world today. Get it on Apple Podcasts, Podomatic, or, from our website:
www.GrowingLoveNetwork.org

My Love Lasts is a 2 to 3 day retreat/seminar that is designed to be flexible in order to meet the needs of your church or organization. For more information go to GrowingLoveNetwork.org

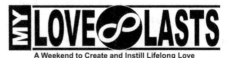

A Weekend to Create and Instill Lifelong Love

growing love network

For Speaking Engagements:
Info@GrowingLoveNetwork.org

For more information:
GrowingLoveNetwork.org